The Making and Meaning
of Hospital Policy
in the United States and Canada

The Making and Meaning
of Hospital Policy
in the United States and Canada

Terry Boychuk

Ann Arbor

THE UNIVERSITY OF MICHIGAN PRESS

2002   2001   2000   1999   4   3   2   1

A CIP catalog record for this book is available from the British Library.

Library of Congress Cataloging-in-Publication Data

Boychuk, Terry, 1964–
    The making and meaning of hospital policy in the United States
   and Canada / Terry Boychuk.
       p.   cm.
    Includes bibliographical references and index.
    ISBN 0-472-10928-6 (alk. paper)
    1. Medical policy—United States—History.   2. Medical
policy—Canada—History.   3. Hospitals—Government policy—United
States—History.   4. Hospitals—Government policy—Canada—History.
I. Title.
RA395.A3.B694   1999
362.1'1'0973—dc21   98-58120
                                                           CIP

Preface

This book endeavors to explain the differing outcomes of political struggles over national health policy in the United States and Canada in the postwar era. More specifically, it is an attempt to account for why hospital politics and policies became driving forces behind the defeat of national health insurance in the United States and the triumph of universal health insurance in Canada. In doing so, this study considers a wider range of historical questions, such as

> why voluntary hospitals, and not government hospitals, came to dominate the hospital industries of the United States and Canada in the late nineteenth and early twentieth centuries;
>
> why state governments lost their definitive role in shaping tax-supported hospital care in the United States before World War II;
>
> why provincial governments directly steered hospital policy in Canada in the prewar era;
>
> why U.S. local governments overwhelmingly allocated public funding for hospital services to municipally owned and operated hospitals;
>
> why Canadian municipalities made voluntary hospitals the primary beneficiaries of local spending on hospital care;
>
> why the United States developed a two-tier hospital system consisting of public hospitals for the poor and private hospitals for those of means;
>
> why Canada called into existence a single-tier hospital system accessible to patients of all social classes;
>
> why Congress, and not the state legislatures, became the singular locus for health reform in the postwar era;
>
> why provincial governments motivated a national policy for universal hospital insurance in Canada;
>
> why U.S. hospital associations opposed universal health insurance, yet became leading advocates for enhancing publicly financed hospital benefits for the poor; and
>
> why Canadian hospital associations cooperated in the formation of mandatory hospital insurance plans.

It is worthwhile to indicate briefly the justification for exploring the historical significance of hospital politics. I began this study with the assumption that the success of political movements to establish national health insurance in North America depended upon overcoming the resistance of the medical profession. If doctors fought the proponents of government-sponsored medical insurance to a standstill, then mandatory hospital insurance would suffer a similar defeat. As I surveyed the history of health policy in the United States and Canada, it became apparent that the evolution of hospital policy could not be deduced from the more dramatic conflicts over publicly financed medical care. To the contrary, incipient arrangements for hospital insurance exerted a disproportionate influence over the development of medical insurance.

Although the American Medical Association surfaced as the most vocal and powerful opponent of national health insurance in the United States, this reactionary stance did not eliminate the prospect of legislative action to ensure access to medical and hospital care for most citizens. Only a private alternative within reach of a majority of Americans would remove consideration of broad-based government insurance from the political agenda. Of its own accord, the medical profession was not inclined to construct a viable substitute for national health insurance. As it was, the hospital industry played an indispensable role in arbitrating the future of American health insurance. In the 1930s, the associated efforts of voluntary hospitals to institutionalize privately financed hospital plans lent ideological and organizational coherence to the postwar expansion of health insurance markets. The hospital-controlled Blue Cross plans transformed the existing foundations of employment-based health insurance, as manifested in U.S. workers' compensation laws, demonstrating to commercial insurers new possibilities for market-based underwriting of health care expenses. Blue Cross also dispelled medical opposition to private insurance while affording U.S. businesses a vehicle for enlarging corporate control over health care finance and for resisting legislative proposals for establishing publicly administered health plans. Hospital insurance anticipated the fate of medical insurance, private and public. When Congress eventually moved to address the needs of Americans disqualified from employment-based insurance in the 1960s, hospital endorsements of government programs for the elderly and poor advanced the cause of national health reform over the objections of the medical profession.

In Canada, federal and provincial governments failed to reach a settlement on national health insurance in the 1940s. Provincial governments then divorced hospital reform from the volatile politics surrounding medical insurance to harness the willingness of Canadian hospitals to embrace progressive legislation. In the late 1940s and early 1950s, some provinces enacted universal hospital plans while other provinces extended the reach of mandatory hospital insurance in various forms. These accomplishments served as a powerful impetus to national legislation aimed at instituting tax-supported hospital insurance in every province. In working out the details of universal hospital insurance in the 1950s, federal legislators assembled a blueprint for medical reform. As national hospital insurance achieved constitutional, fiscal, and administrative integrity, as well as enjoying popular acclaim, the political barriers to federal sponsorship of a nationwide system of medical insurance diminished considerably. Universal medical insurance, as enacted in the 1960s, duplicated the principles and practices of the national program for hospital insurance.

Voluntary hospitals formed the nucleus of the U.S. and Canadian hospital industries and determined the political outlooks of their respective trade associations. Notwithstanding this important similarity, U.S. and Canadian hospital associations revealed differing ideological tendencies that frustrated, or otherwise advanced, the cause of national health insurance. U.S. hospital associations never wavered in their efforts to preempt government-sponsored hospital insurance for the gainfully employed. U.S. hospitals demonstrated formidable skill in arranging a legal, administrative, and economic basis for private hospital insurance. That same prowess found equal expression in their successful bid to limit the scope of publicly financed hospital benefits to the poor and to make voluntary hospitals beneficiaries of new sources of public funding for hospital care. By contrast, Canadian hospitals did not dispute the objective of universal hospital insurance. Some differences of opinion appeared among hospitals on the ways and means of achieving comprehensive coverage. But the notions held sway that Canadian governments had the right and obligation to ensure universal access to hospital care and that mandatory hospital insurance was a practical necessity.

One starting point for arriving at an informed understanding of why national health policy traveled separate paths in each country is a detailed account of how U.S. and Canadian hospitals constructed their interests. Why did the U.S. hospital industry generate political ideologies and strategies that rendered extremely difficult any movement toward national health insurance? Why was the converse apparent in Canada? A considered answer to these questions would examine state, provincial, and local policies and how they informed the vocations of U.S. and Canadian hospitals. Although charitable corporations identified with specific religious, ethnic, and linguistic groups came to own and operate most hospitals in the United States and Canada, hospital endeavors were not exclusively a matter of private initiative. Since colonial times, regional governments played continuous and significant roles, albeit variable ones, in arranging institutional care for the sick. Hospital pursuits have been an admixture of public and private enterprise from the very beginning. And so, the point of departure for this study is the evolution of state, provincial, and local policies governing hospital ventures in the prewar era. Nineteenth- and early twentieth-century political movements in the United States and Canada mobilized specific biases in hospital policy. The organizations, professions, and lobbies implicated in those antecedent policies constituted the political environment in which federal legislators set out to discover the appropriate ends and means of national health reform. The historical practices and meanings of government-sponsored hospital care greatly differed between the two countries.

In the United States, myriad forces conspired to prompt state legislatures to delegate control over publicly financed hospital care to local governments. Local experiments converged on one dominant pattern in the late nineteenth and early twentieth centuries: public spending on municipal hospitals expressly built and maintained for the poor. The identification of government hospitals with the poverty-stricken, coupled with the dramatic growth of voluntary hospitals attending to the self-supporting, informed U.S. thinking about public and private responsibilities for financing and managing hospital care. The prevailing view held that extending government sovereignty over hospital care beyond that needed to provide for the poor threatened private enterprise and initiative, jeopardized standards of care, and endangered scientific and technological progress. U.S. hospital associations and state legislators remained loyal to these precepts and worked at cross-purposes with national advocates of universal health insurance. Congress affirmed those understandings of the public interest in hospital care: government programs would specifically address the needs of those excluded from the private economy of health care.

In Canada, the provinces adopted laws that called for open admissions to all voluntary and municipal hospitals and that obliged provincial and local governments to compensate hospitals for the expense of caring for patients who could not afford all or part of the costs of their treatment. These mandatory subsidies were perceived as a mechanism for assisting local initiative, enforcing high standards of operation, encouraging patterns of hospital ownership that mirrored the social diversity of Canada, stabilizing hospital budgets, and releasing hospitals from the constraints of revenues derived from fees and endowments. These positive attributes of government financing and supervision appeared as corollaries of the transparent maxim of prewar hospital policy: universal access to essential hospital services. Provincial legislators and hospital associations, through example and advocacy, successfully made equity the imperative of national hospital policy.

The empirical evidence presented in this study comes from varied sources. The postwar evolution of health policy in the United States and Canada has been well documented and interpreted from a variety of perspectives in the secondary literature. From them, I first gathered insight into the general contours of national policy making in both countries. Where my own primary research has confirmed the arguments of several accomplished historians of health policy, I have gladly relied upon them and cited them repeatedly. Where primary sources have indicated significant departures from the established historiography or uncovered previously overlooked evidence, I directly cite legislative digests, legislative debates, statements from interested lobbies in several forums, including publicly and privately arranged inquiries, hearings, commissions, and so on. The historiography of prewar hospital policy is much less developed than general histories of state, provincial, and local governments in North America. Here, I have often drawn upon government documents to reconstruct the dynamics of hospital financing, organization, and policy. This is most apparent in the case studies of New York State, New York City, and the Province of Ontario in the first half of the book.

Before introducing the broader theoretical arguments concerning the development of hospital policy in the United States and Canada, the methodological underpinnings of this research require some elaboration. This book adopts a comparative and historical methodology to frame the analysis of policy making in North America. The intent of the comparative method is not to arrive at an exhaustive interpretation of the differing outcomes of national policy making in the postwar era. An argument of that scope would examine any or all historical events of some conceivable bearing on the formation of national legislation. Rather, the express purpose of this study is to identify a relatively few, distinctive historical processes that yield the greatest amount of explanatory leverage over the unsettled questions marked for deliberation here.

This study observes Seymour Martin Lipset's counsel that "knowledge of Canada or the United States is the best way to gain insight into the other North American country" (1990, xii). The comparative method is most instructive when applied to understanding differences between societies otherwise following broadly similar lines of historical development, as with the United States and Canada. Comparisons of like countries simplify the task of identifying historical differences responsible for other cross-national variations. Also, the fewer the differences, the more likely they matter. U.S.-Canadian contrasts produce much more confidence in evaluating the causal weight of varying historical antecedents to national health reform than comparing North American societies to other nations with profoundly dissimilar social and political histories. The latter comparisons imply so many discrepancies of potential causal significance that they render extremely doubtful the task of assigning relative explanatory importance to any one of them.

The purpose of this study is not to establish a general statement about the historical origins of national health insurance beyond the U.S. and Canadian cases. There are many paths to national health insurance as is apparent among the advanced industrial democracies. European contrasts have generally informed comparative studies seeking to account for the unique qualities of the U.S. welfare state. Several students of health policy have drawn insights from this diverse scholarship to call attention to the distinctive aspects of U.S. society and politics that inhibited, or precluded altogether, the adoption of national health insurance. If the question is why the United States did not follow the social democratic or corporatist routes to national health insurance demonstrated in Europe, then we have promising answers. If the question is why the United States did not discover another avenue, a liberal democratic one, then we have much less convincing answers. The classical European routes were also closed to Canada. The liberal democratic institutions of the United States find close parallels in Canada. U.S.-Canadian comparisons constitute a logical starting point for identifying the specific elements of the U.S. political tradition that militated against national health insurance and, correspondingly, for bringing into sharp relief those properties of Canada's liberal democratic synthesis that advanced the cause of national health insurance.

While the motivation of this research is to seek out telling differences, it is also important to mention a few telling likenesses of national politics in the United States and Canada. Since the common attributes of each country do not enter into the analysis as decisive factors, I want to make explicit here what remains implicit in the elaboration of the book's central arguments. Two singularities of North American political development provide the backdrop for the theoretical statements offered in this study and merit immediate consideration: first, party dominance over policy formation; and second, the relative influence of class-based political mobilization.

U.S. and Canadian polities democratized before they bureaucratized. The early extension of the franchise confirmed legislatures and political parties as the dominant institutions of national policy making. Colonial administrations in North America offered no pretext for the emergence of bureaucratic government. Patronage-oriented parties became the locus of policy formation in the nineteenth century. Civil service reforms aimed at professionalizing public administration came late in the nineteenth and early twentieth centuries and were badly compromised in their design and application. Even as U.S. and Canadian legislators instituted more bureaucratic-like administration, they did so in ways that jealously guarded their policy-making initiative and power. The administrative branches of government have ultimately exerted much less influence over health policy than the legislative branches in the historical periods scrutinized in this study.

If parties and parliamentarians arbitrated the fate of national health insurance, then it would be appropriate to give some definition to the general contours of party politics in North America. Here, too, striking parallels characterized party formation in the United States and Canada. The granting of the vote to the laboring classes in early stages of industrialization dampened working-class radicalism. Labor movements could not appeal to the solidarities implied in the shared experience of political disenfranchisement as was typical of European workers. Pronounced barriers to working-class political mobilization stemming from crosscutting social cleavages also contributed to the hegemony of loosely articulated bourgeois parties over national policy making. The reconstitution of labor movements during the depression and their subsequent incorporation into national politics as formidable allies of progressive legislation were important moments in the reconstruction of social policy in both countries. Nonetheless, class-specific appeals did not become the central organizing theme of national campaigns in the postwar era. Class-based politics supplemented, but did not supplant, those ethnic, racial, religious, linguistic, and regional identities already woven into the fabric of the national parties.

The fate of national health insurance did not reflect the success or failure of the left. The social democratic delegations to the national legislatures—the liberal wing of the Democratic party in the United States and the Cooperative Commonwealth Federation in Canada—did not command parliamentary majorities in the postwar era. Legislators from the center and the right of the political spectrum cast the deciding votes. The area of agreement spanning the major parties governed national policy making. What differentiated the United States from Canada was the nature of that consensus. Bipartisan agreement confirmed private insurance as the vehicle for mass coverage in the United States. This same accord reserved for government the role of insurer of last resort for those disqualified from employer-financed health plans. In Canada, a coalition of provincial governments of every political stripe—Liberal, CCF, Progressive Conservative, and Social Credit—launched a campaign for national hospital insurance in the 1950s. The federal response, grants-in-aid of universal hospital plans under provincial direction, received the endorsement of every party represented in the House of Commons. Yet another cross-party alliance, this time a Liberal–New Democrat coalition government, added medical services to the federal government's health insurance portfolio in the 1960s.

This study does not try to account for the specific roles that political parties have played in the elaboration of hospital policies. Rather, it is an attempt to understand the historical origins of the prevailing conceptions of the public interest in hospital care that transcended party divisions and prompted U.S. and Canadian legislators to establish very different arrangements for hospital insurance in the postwar era. Those perceptions not only spanned party lines, they reached across several tiers of government and informed the political behavior of interest groups arising out of the health care industries of the United States and Canada.

As detailed in chapter 1, the theoretical arguments guiding this research draw inspiration from institutionalist approaches to clarifying the origins of policy making. The perspective adopted in this book calls attention to the socially constructed logics of policy making: institutionalized sets of beliefs, values, and norms that define the legitimate scope of government action within specific policy domains. The second insight drawn from institutional analysis concerns how policy making generates reciprocal influences between socioeconomic and political realms. Politically mobilized constituencies arising from civil society perpetually create, reaffirm, reform, or dismantle the institutions of government. An institutionalist approach also considers the ways in which legislative conventions reshape civil society in deliberate and unanticipated ways and, thus, mediate the articulation of demands in the political sphere.

Chapters 2 and 3 compare and contrast the social and political origins of American and Canadian hospital charities from colonial times to the Great Depression. They highlight the common features of hospital development in both countries, namely, how religious cleavages generated a permissive context for the proliferation of voluntary hospitals in the nineteenth and early twentieth centuries. Correspondingly, government hospitals did not become the principal means for rendering institutional care for the sick in North America. Hospital development in the United States and that in Canada also resembled one another with respect to the commercial transformation of hospital charities in the late nineteenth century. Nursing reform, urbanization, and the incorporation of medical care into the hospital interior extended the appeal of hospital care to the generality of sick persons, rich and poor alike, but under a new commercial ethos. Fees, rather than donations, constituted the single largest source of income for acute-care hospitals in North America at the turn of the century. Another similarity concerned the plight of the poor and public financing of hospital enterprises. As voluntary hospitals tailored their services to patients of means, arranging hospital care for the poor became an indivisible responsibility of government. Whereas public and private charity had previously shared the burdens of caring for the sick poor, these expenses were increasingly drawn against government accounts in the closing decades of the nineteenth century.

Emergent patterns of government spending, however, constituted the signal difference between the two countries. U.S. and Canadian governments formulated discrepant strategies for underwriting hospital charity within the larger context of the new hospital economy. These policies mediated the commercial transformation of hospital care. Hospital policy in the United States promoted separate hospitals and different standards of care for poorer and wealthier Americans. Canadian law stipulated universal access to all hospitals and promoted common standards of care for patients of all classes.

Chapter 2 seeks to identify and explain the historical dynamics of Canadian hospital policy. In meeting the most compelling challenge of nineteenth-century poor relief in Canada—the management of immigrant traffic—provincial governments set the legislative precedents for modern hospital policy. The provinces decided against building and operating institutions for the sick, and they neither required nor encouraged local governments to establish their own hospitals. In lieu of government provision, the provinces delegated hospital initiatives to voluntary associations wherever possible, leading to the development of a network of locally autonomous hospitals primarily identified with Canada's Protestant and Catholic churches. The settling of the hospitals issue was part of a grander political compromise leading to the formation of a semipublic, semiprivate charitable establishment. This chapter also explores how provincial governments reworked the laws compensating private charities for seeing to the hospital needs of the poor. Canadian hospital policies likened hospital charities to public utilities, entitled to government subsidies, both provincial and municipal, and subject to provincial regulation. Mandatory spending on hospital charity cemented a cooperative public-private alliance that differentiated Canadian hospital endeavors from those of the United States. Provincial legislation called into existence an egalitarian, single-tier hospital system of voluntary and municipal hospitals, defined in law as public hospitals: open to all on the basis of medical need.

Chapter 3 explores the complex political origins of the United States' public and private hospital systems. The concerns here are the privatization of voluntary hospital charities in the mid–nineteenth century and the calculus of local politics that favored public investments in municipal hospitals for the poor. Instead of legalizing hospital undertakings as joint public-private ventures, state constitutions divided hospital charities, as with many other branches of the U.S. philanthropic establishment, into two self-governing branches, one private, the other public. Private hospitals formally emerged at midcentury with the reworking of state constitutions and with accumulation of case law voiding state funding and regulation of business corporations. Voluntary hospitals were left to finance and manage themselves without state supervision. With few exceptions, the states delegated public initiatives in the realm of hospital care to local governments. This partitioning of hospital projects among the municipalities and private charities precluded egalitarianism from becoming the ascendant motive of U.S. hospital policy. Local hospital policies absented most voluntary institutions from publicly financed arrangements for hospital charity. The widespread construction of municipal hospitals for the poor coincided with the commercial transformation of private hospitals in the late nineteenth century to institutionalize a two-tier hospital industry in the United States.

The second part of the book follows the differing trajectories of hospital policy in the United States and Canada from the onset of the depression to the 1960s. The changing hospital economy prompted the reconstruction of hospital policy in both countries. Hospital fees in the early decades of the twentieth century consistently rose faster than the wages of working- and middle-class patients, making a second transformation of hospital finance a virtual necessity. The depression added urgency to public and private efforts to establish a framework for hospital insurance in North America. Even so, the stringencies of the 1930s differed for U.S. and Canadian hospitals and engendered distinctive political responses. The contrasting influences were the fixed patterns of public spending on hospital care. Government subsidies stabilized the finances of all voluntary and municipal hospitals in Canada's public hospital system. U.S. conventions limited public spending to government hospitals. This did little to mitigate the hardships of voluntary hospitals and prompted fears that the expanding public sector might eclipse the private hospital economy. Whereas Canadian hospitals subsequently cooperated in the formation of legislation converting hospital subsidies into public hospital insurance, in the United States voluntary hospitals envisaged private insurance as the means to preempt any further extensions of government sovereignty over hospital financing and management.

Chapter 4 follows the circuitous path to universal hospital insurance in Canada. In the 1940s, federal committees brokered an agreement with representatives of the health care establishment on the design of a national health plan. This accord found its demise in federal-provincial disagreements over national fiscal policy. The distinguishing feature of health reform in Canada was that the federal government had no apparent constitutional warrant to legislate a national program for health insurance apart from the general consent of the provincial governments. Subsequently, the initiative passed from the federal government to the provinces. In the 1950s, a coalition of provincial governments did eventually surface to reinstate a federal commitment to hospital reform. Ottawa then laid the cornerstone of national health insurance with grants-in-aid of universal hospital plans in every province. The emergent consensus was that the second transformation of hospital finance—the transition from direct payments for hospital fees to insurance-based reimbursements—should conform to the principle underlying the first one: universal access to hospital care.

Chapter 5 bears witness to the incipient primacy of the American Hospital Association and Congress in the remaking of U.S. hospital policy in the postwar era. Whereas provincial forces arbitrated national hospital reform in Canada, state governments and state hospital associations mostly found themselves on the receiving end of policies articulated in Washington, DC. The American Hospital Association became the national sponsor for the private insurance movement and then formed one of the pillars of the vigorous opposition to national health insurance. Federal legislators correspondingly declined any obligations to underwrite hospital care for the working population. What remained to be seen was how Congress would reconstruct publicly financed health benefits for those stranded from employment-based insurance. Federal policies enacted in the 1940s and 1950s hastened the decomposition of traditional methods for bringing hospital care to the poor, namely, tax-supported municipal hospitals. As private hospitals increasingly became liable for the care of uninsured and underinsured patients, the American Hospital Association and the financial arm of the voluntary hospitals, the Blue Cross Association, emerged as leading proponents of federal subsidies to private hospitals for the care of public dependents. Congress responded with the enactment of Medicare and Medicaid programs. The advent of government-financed hospital insurance for old-age pensioners and public assistance recipients validated the historical precepts of U.S. hospital policy: public arrangements for the poor and private arrangements for the self-supporting.

This book would have been impossible without the contributions of many philanthropic individuals and institutions. The Program on Non-Profit Organizations at Yale University underwrote my preliminary research into the political and legal history of U.S. and Canadian hospitals. Several organizations at Princeton University provided critical financial assistance for the archival research needed to complete this study. They include the Association of Princeton Graduate Alumni, the Council on Regional Studies, the Center of International Studies, the Center of Domestic and Comparative Policy, and the Princeton Society of Fellows of the

Woodrow Wilson Foundation. I am obliged to the skillful archivists at the Provincial Archives of British Columbia, Ontario, and Saskatchewan and at the National Archives of Canada for their interest and assistance, as I am to the staff at the American Hospital Association library and archive who generously gave of their time and expertise.

I owe a considerable debt to my former mentors in the Department of Sociology at Princeton University. Paul DiMaggio, Gene Burns, Michele Lamont, Howard Taylor, Walter Wallace, Robert Wuthnow, and Viviana Zelizer have all profoundly shaped my understanding of the sociological enterprise. I am uniquely indebted to Frank Dobbin and Paul Starr. Frank Dobbin has been as brilliant a mentor, collaborator, and friend as one could ever hope to have. Paul Starr's contributions to the social history of U.S. health care inspired this study, and his personal interest and faith in the project did much to sustain my confidence in the merits of the research.

Several people have kindly read some or all of the chapters and offered helpful comments for revision over the years or in other ways prompted me to reconsider and refine the defining arguments of the book. I would particularly like to thank Bradford Gray, Bai Gao, Peter Dobkin Hall, Mary Ellen Hollingsworth, Tom Janoski, Patrice Leclerc, Antonia Maioni, John Meyer, Steven Rathgeb Smith, Robert Sprinkle, Malcolm G. Taylor, John Thompson, and Patricia Thornton. I would also like to thank Rebecca McDermott of the University of Michigan Press for her patience and tireless efforts to bring the book to press. And last, but not least of all, I extend my appreciation to Jackie Walcome and Aldo Hertz for unfailing encouragement throughout the final revisions of the manuscript.

Contents

Tables

CHAPTER 1

The Social and Political Origins of Hospital Policy

In the 1940s, the federal governments of the United States and Canada deliberated, and failed to legislate, national health insurance. In each country, federal legislators temporized with labor and tax laws favoring the development of privately financed, employment-based health insurance as a more general alternative to social insurance. As the limits of voluntary insurance became clearly visible in the 1950s and 1960s, both countries were forced to confront the realities of market-based health plans. Hospitals, doctors, workers, employers, and private insurers could not arrange universal access to health benefits as contractual parties, even if governments subsidized the health care expenses of the poorest and most frail citizens. Health politics reverted to consideration of government-mandated coverage for some, most, or all of the population. At stake was a dramatic, unprecedented expansion of federal authority over health care finance that had been previously considered and dismissed as politically unfeasible.

Federal legislators in each country responded quite differently to the dilemma of health reform. In the United States, Congress patiently waited for market-based health insurance to demonstrate its full potential before establishing tax-supported hospital and medical insurance for those Americans unambiguously excluded from employer-sponsored health plans, namely, the aged and the poor. The resulting programs—Medicare for pensioners and Medicaid for means-tested recipients of public assistance—have served as the benchmarks for U.S. health policy since their inception in 1965. National health reform exhibited a central preoccupation with establishing a clear division of labor between private and public insurance, even at the painful expense of barring a significant minority of Americans from coverage of either kind. Tax-supported health insurance primarily extended to individuals defined in federal and state laws as qualified beneficiaries of income-maintenance programs. Voluntary insurance extended to those defined as gainfully employed and largely depended upon their employers' willingness to subsidize their enrollment in group insurance. Most workers did obtain some private coverage, and a smaller number did not. The others caught in the abyss between public and private insurance were the unemployed. The enduring presence of the noninsured and underinsured was the regrettable, but necessary, trade-off for upholding what was perceived as a greater good. To U.S. legislators, the public interest was best served by fragmenting and dispersing responsibility for health care financing among governments, health care providers, private insurers, employers, and workers. In Canada, federal legislators opted for universal, compulsory health insurance at the reluctant expense of abolishing voluntary health plans. National legislation effectively dismantled private hospital insurance in 1957 and private medical insurance in 1967. By 1971, every province had reconstituted hospital and medical insurance under direct public administration with grants-in-aid from the federal government. Federal contributions to the provincial health plans stipulated comprehensive coverage of all necessary hospital and medical care, available to all citizens on uniform terms and conditions.

This book endeavors to account for why U.S. and Canadian legislators made these differing choices as they reconstructed publicly sponsored health care in the postwar era. Why did U.S. reforms attach surpassing importance to differentiating the realms of public insurance from private insurance? Why did universalism become the controlling motive of Canadian reforms?

This study takes the historical emergence of hospital policy as its point of departure. The reason for underscoring its significance stems from one empirical observation. In each country, the vast majority of public expenditures on personal health services went to acute-care hospitals in the prewar era. Medical care, insofar as it could be classified as tax supported, was mostly incidental to publicly arranged hospital care. From colonial times to World War II, civilian hospitals fell under the legislative jurisdiction of state, provincial, and local governments. Long before the arrival of federal interest in hospital finance, these governments had elaborated statutory law specifically regulating hospital endeavors. Constitutional and common law also defined the legitimate ends and means of tax-supported hospital care, the scope of private prerogatives over hospital financing and management, and the relationship between them. There were no comparable arrangements for medical care. This historical sequencing made hospital policy the avant-garde of political efforts to convert health care finance to the medium of insurance in the postwar era.

U.S. and Canadian legislators moved more boldly and with greater clarity of purpose on hospital reforms than on public policies devoted to initiating lawful arrangements for prepaid medical care. Adaptations to hospital policy generally came earlier, with greater ease, and exerted a larger influence over the broader architecture of health insurance. In the United States, the hospital associations and state legislators quietly issued legal warrants for employment-based health plans. Medical associations would eventually become the most vociferous defenders of voluntary insurance in political forums. The American Hospital Association and its insurance subsidiary, the Blue Cross Association, settled with federal officials the terms of compulsory hospital insurance in the 1960s. Medical lobbies led the faltering opposition to national health reform. In Canada, the hospital associations magnanimously consented to universal coverage in deliberations with provincial premiers over the scope of public hospital insurance. These accords provided the foundations for national hospital legislation in the 1950s. And, the success of universal hospital insurance handed to federal legislators a politically popular and constitutionally robust model for enacting national medical insurance in the 1960s.

This book argues that the historical formation of hospital industries in the United States and Canada lent themselves to the emergence of two distinctive sorts of political rationality. I refer to these socially constructed logics of policy making as policy paradigms (Hall 1993). In both countries, the paradigms governing hospital policy emerged in the postbellum era. They were the unintended and unforeseen consequences of antebellum laws regulating U.S. and Canadian hospital charities. Only later did legislators and hospital associations derive coherent ideologies from these arrangements. They did so as the hospitals were making the transition from relatively undifferentiated agents of poor relief to special-purpose institutions devoted to therapeutic advances in nursing and medical care. This transformation coincided with the commercialization of hospital finance and the rise of political movements bent on rationalizing policy making and policy implementation. The resulting political thrusts converged on clarifying the parameters of hospital policy and on constructing doctrinal justifications for them. These paradigms served as conceptual templates for national health reform in the postwar era. In short, the U.S. paradigm had historically indicated separate hospital accommodations for the self-supporting and public dependents: private arrangements for the former and public arrangements for the latter. By contrast, the Canadian paradigm acknowledged no such social or economic distinctions, and it designated provincial governments as guarantors of universal access to hospital care. These opposing notions of the public interest in hospital care ultimately served as the cornerstones of two very different systems of health insurance.

An Institutionalist Perspective on Policy Making and Political Rationality

This study draws upon the theoretical rubrics of the new institutionalism in the social sciences (March and Olsen 1989; DiMaggio and Powell 1991). The claim made on behalf of this approach is that it can better account for the observed configurations of political mobilization, for the behavior of legislative bodies, and for the blending of these phenomena in the making and remaking of hospital policy in the United States and Canada.

Three insights guide institutionalist perspectives on policy making. First, policy making is a historically informed process (Thelen and Steinmo 1992). Although policy making is ultimately concerned with responding to, or inducing, social and political change, it begins from historical experience. Second, historical experience is grounded in social relations. Institutions—as they consist of established rules, regulations, and practices—pattern social interaction. Institutional environments have political and socioeconomic referents. The former concern the universe of conventions expressed in law and enforced through coercive reserves of the state. The latter arise out of formally voluntary agreements among consenting individuals and organizations. These institutional environments mediate policy making. They constrain the actions and intentions of groups implicated in legislative deliberation and, thus, generate continuities between preexisting and emergent law. An institutionalist account of policy making also draws attention to how the organizational dynamics of state and civil society interact over time and mutually reshape each other in anticipated and unforeseen ways (Hall 1986, 3–22; Skocpol 1992, 41–60). Third, institutions are mediums of cultural expression. It is through institutions that meaning and understanding become shared and reproduced (Berger and Luckmann 1966). Consequently, institutions constrain as they empower. The cultural scripts embedded in institutions provide ideological sanction for experimenting with new practices and for transforming existing ones.

The Making of Policy

Policy making is most often described as the outcome of political processes that govern the ways in which policies are decided as opposed to the substantive outcomes of policy making. These processes consist of institutionalized roles, norms, and expectations that pattern the relationships between incumbents of political office and mobilized groups that seek to influence policy. In liberal democratic polities such as the United States and Canada, legislative conventions cast policy makers in the role of impartial conciliators. In this specific sense, it is not deemed legitimate for officeholders to interfere with the formation of politically active associations arising out of civil society. Legislators are also expected to grant interested lobbies the broadest latitude in articulating their political demands. Legislative priorities subsequently emerge as officeholders arbitrate conflicts of interest between politically organized groups. Optimal policies are those that satisfy the demands of as many interest groups as possible, even if biased in favor of specific groups thought to command superior political resources. Thus the outcomes of policy making can be directly attributed to the generation of ideologies and interests from social collectivities not implicated in the formal apparatus of government. A description of the coalitions that interest groups have established, or failed to establish, with other mobilized groups would ostensibly complete this account of how political forces emanating from civil society inform policy making.

There is a relatively straightforward explanation of national hospital reform that can be drawn from liberal-pluralist interpretations of policy making. In the United States, the national hospital associations opposed universal hospital insurance. They became founding members of an impressive political coalition bent on institutionalizing privately financed, employment-based hospital insurance. This alliance consisted of some of the most economically powerful groups in U.S. society—the medical profession, the industrial establishment, and private insurance concerns. In Canada, the hospital associations allied with provincial governments in the making of universal hospital insurance. The hospitals made no pronounced effort to assemble a grand political consortium with doctors, business, and insurers locked together in defense of voluntary insurance. U.S. political hostility to national hospital insurance greatly surpassed that of Canada. The view that interest group politics determined the outcomes of national reform provides a roughly accurate portrayal of how these policy battles were waged and won in both countries. However, the principal weakness of focusing on the minutia of political jostling is to mistake the actors for the drama. Left unanswered is the more fundamental question of why hospitals constructed their interests as they did. This problem is particularly acute when one considers the different political fates of U.S. and Canadian hospitals. In each country, the social and economic dynamics of hospital development were remarkably similar as will become apparent hereafter. In sum, the political origins of postwar reforms cannot be uniquely attributed to the social origins of the North American hospital industries.

The perspective advanced here expands upon the insights drawn from interpretations of policy making that privilege the social origins of political behavior. Bringing institutional variables into the analysis renders a more informed account of why politically mobilized groups chose their policy preferences as they did. This involves acknowledging the historical antecedents of interest group formation that derive from the preexisting legal order. Understanding how hospital associations discovered their interests necessarily draws attention to the intermediate role of government. All corporate entities, hospitals included, operate within frameworks created, sustained, and altered through lawmaking. Interest groups do not articulate political preferences as the unmediated expression of their constituents' motives, if such convictions are thought of as existentially prior to politics, policy, and law. All legal systems create taxonomies of permissible institutional forms, practices, and objectives, withholding specific designs from some corporations while prescribing them for others. In each country, the respective hospital lobbies emerged after the legal status of hospital charities had been decided in the nineteenth and early twentieth centuries. Constitutional, statutory, and common law entrusted various private, semipublic, and public functions to hospital governing boards. In the United States, these functions were more private. In Canada, they were more public. These earlier grants of authority proved to be critical factors in shaping the collective interpretation of hospital ambitions in the mid–twentieth century. They were as important as the social and economic transformations of hospital endeavors in the late nineteenth century: the reconstruction of the hospital-based professions; the rapid commercialization of hospital finance; and the extension of hospital services to the respectable classes.

A second departure from conventional liberal-pluralist interpretations of policy making highlighted in this study is a respecification of the role of legislators in policy formation that calls attention to the fundamental duality of political office holding. The defining characteristic of legislators is that they are situated in the boundary between the institutions of government and of civil society. Legislative behavior is doubly regulated. In one instance, policymakers come to occupy positions within the formal apparatus of government representing, and responsible to, political associations stemming from civil society. In other instance, legislators exercise control over society in accordance with mandates embedded in the historical accretion of constitutional and statutory law. Legislators are empowered to change the law as warranted, but they are also sworn to uphold the spirit and letter of law as they find it. Just as politically mobilized groups seek to inform legislators' perceptions of the appropriate objects of policy making, previously institutionalized practices of government also normalize and reinforce policymakers' understandings of the public interest. These latter understandings may not be susceptible to fundamental restatement except through extraordinary forms of political mobilization.

Historically, lawmaking is constitutive of both socioeconomic and governmental realms, and hospital care was not the monopoly of private corporations in the nineteenth-century United States and Canada. In each country, political movements vested governments with specific forms of responsibility over hospital care in constitutional and statutory law, just as they defined the legal purposes, uses, and limits of private prerogative over the institutional care of the sick. In each realm, these legal innovations outlived the political coalitions responsible for calling them into existence and developed a force and meaning apart from the hopes and aspirations of their original sponsors. In the late nineteenth century, the social transformation of hospital care precipitated a reinterpretation of the laws governing public financing of hospital charity. These laws gathered new ideological loadings as they became further ensconced in the political order. The subsequent refinement of hospital law created highly institutionalized sets of principles and practices accorded to public authority over hospital care. These routinized meanings formed the second intermediary bridging prewar hospital policy and postwar hospital reform.

Thus, the analysis put forth here emphasizes the two institutional legacies of the prewar legal order that prefaced national health reform. The first was the institutionalization of private privileges and obligations in the realm of hospital care. The second concerned the legally sanctioned forms of public authority over hospital endeavors. How did these legacies inform postwar policy making? Both countries dramatically reconstructed the ways and means of hospital financing, public and private, with the arrival of federal interventions in health policy. What remained constant were the antecedent purposes of prewar hospital policy. In each country, historical allocations of public and private sovereignty over hospital care constituted paradigms for national hospital reform. They formed the historical basis of a coherent set of meanings that both constrained and enabled innovations in hospital policy. These understandings limited the range of possibilities that hospital lobbies and policymakers considered desirable legislative avenues for reconstructing hospital finance. At the same time, these paradigms afforded legislators and the hospital associations legitimate grounds for testing untried methods of insuring hospital care, for evaluating their appropriateness, and ultimately, for entrenching very different kinds of health insurance regimes in the United States and Canada.

The Meaning of Policy

The concept of policy paradigms originates in the writings of Thomas Kuhn (1970) and reformulations by Peter Hall (1993) and Frank Dobbin (1994). This approach likens policy paradigms to Kuhn's notion of scientific paradigms as problem-solving heuristics. Policy paradigms encompass propositions about the nature of political processes, taken-for-granted assumptions about the appropriate objects of government action, and models of what policymakers are likely to perceive as social problems requiring public solutions. Legislators choose among competing policy alternatives in highly scripted ways because policy paradigms provide them with ideological justifications and rationales for pursuing some objectives and not others. They acquit policymakers for creating fiscal and administrative capacities that governments did not formerly possess and excuse lawmakers for destroying existing instruments of rule insofar as new policy reaffirms the canons of antecedent policy.

Policy paradigms entail generative and transformative potential. Whereas some accounts of policy making identify cultural influences as sources of policy inertia and attribute policy dynamism to the clash of interests, the perspective suggested here stresses the driving force of ideology. Policy paradigms resemble cultural tool kits for coping with problems of adjustment stemming from social change (Swidler 1986). All institutions must adapt to changing environments so as to preserve their raison d'être. Policies, too, need to change in order to stay the same: continuity of purpose also begets innovation. The implication is that policy paradigms are compatible with, and manifest themselves in, a range of practices over time. In the United States, the governmental imperative of providing refuge to those excluded from the commerce of hospital care has appeared in several overlapping guises: local poor-law hospitals at first; federal subsidies of private hospital construction in a later era; and social insurance and reformed public assistance programs in most recent times. In Canada, the public interest in maintaining universal access to hospital care assumed several forms: provincial subsidies to hospital charities initially; the addition of mandated local spending in another period; and finally, joint federal-provincial financing of compulsory hospital insurance.

A no less important corollary of how policy paradigms construct the political order is the way in which they constitute the social order. Policy paradigms also encompass propositions about the nature of civil society insofar as drawing distinctions between public and private spheres of action is an inescapable component of policy making. These distinctions contain implicit and explicit notions about which problems are more appropriately addressed with private solutions. As with legislators, policy paradigms afford politically mobilized groups ideological motivations for backing some policies and not others. These socially constructed logics of private privilege condition interest group prospects for setting the direction of policy innovation. U.S. and Canadian paradigms historically ascribed differing institutional identities to hospital corporations. Antecedent hospital policy engendered dissimilar policy-oriented terminologies and demands from the hospital associations in each country. In the United States, hospital lobbies entered into political frays over postwar health reform sporting a vocabulary for describing and legitimating private financing of hospital benefits for the working population, for denouncing public sovereignty over health insurance for the employed, and for promoting government programs for those exiled from commercial insurance. In Canada, the political glossary of the hospital associations contained much more generous expressions for describing the role of government in hospital finance even as it underscored the importance of private prerogative over hospital management.

The remaining sections of this chapter provide a brief overview of the development of U.S. and Canadian hospital industries and the evolution of hospital policy from colonial times to the postwar era. The discussion begins with the social origins of hospital charities in the nineteenth and early twentieth centuries. In each country, denominational rivalries intersected with commercial opportunities to place voluntary, nonprofit corporations at the forefront of hospital enterprises. The concluding arguments draw attention to the similarities and differences that marked the long-run formation of U.S. and Canadian polities. The affinities were evident in the historical sequencing of political reforms. Taking colonial forms of government as their starting point, Americans and Canadians reconstructed the procedural foundations of policy making in three successive periods. The antebellum era confirmed political parties and legislatures as the dominant institutions of policy formation. In the postbellum era, reform movements channeled legislative partisanship in the direction of programmatic initiative. And last, the remaking of federalism to accommodate a national presence in the hospital policy also brought with it new departures in the frameworks for setting policy. Considering these broader parallels provides the occasion for identifying the decisive historical variations in policy making that brought forward opposing versions of health reform in the postwar era.

The Social Origins and Transformation of Hospital Charity

The social and economic dynamics of hospital development in the United States and Canada closely approximated each other. The present discussion draws attention to those aspects uniting the evolution of the North American hospital industries: the early association of hospital enterprises with charitable purposes; the subsequent emergence of commercial and secular influences over hospital financing and management and, correspondingly, how these innovations popularized demand for hospital care;

the commanding heights reserved for private charities during the rapid growth of the hospital industry in the late nineteenth century; and finally, those aspects of the common law that facilitated the transformation of hospital charities into their distinctly modern form. Accounting for these similarities provides a context for isolating the historical factors that differentiated hospital policy from one country to another.

A description of nineteenth-century hospital charity must precede any discussion of the subsequent evolution of U.S. and Canadian hospital industries. Confessionally based associations, churches, religious orders, and local governments founded and managed hospitals in North America. These hospitals were not commercial enterprises as twentieth-century observers came to know them. Hospitals labored within the strictest and most commonly understood meaning of charity—the relief of poverty. Fees paled in comparison to income from private donations and governmental appropriations since the risk of hospital-transmitted fevers and infections had previously kept all but the most destitute from seeking shelter in hospitals. The family remained the primary guardian of health in the nineteenth century, and hospitals could not best the care of supportive relatives. Hospitals generally catered to friendless immigrants or to others whose kinship networks were denied them in periods of illness.

A midcentury reform movement endeavored to redefine hospitals as curative, as opposed to palliative, institutions. Britain's Florence Nightingale initiated an energetic program for hospital modernization that swept across the United States and Canada: the professionalization of nursing; administrative reorganization; the redesign of hospital architecture; and the associated adoption of vastly improved hygienic practices. These reforms gradually dissolved the hospital's reputation as an antechamber to the grave (Rosenberg 1987). At the same time, urbanization began to lessen individuals' reliance upon kin for nursing in times of sickness and, thus, wrought unprecedented demands for institutional care outside of the orbit of the household. And last, advances in surgery and other diagnostic technologies made hospital care an indispensable component of medical practice (Starr 1982).

The therapeutic revolution in hospital services begat other transformations in the late nineteenth and early twentieth centuries—one cultural and the other commercial. Access to hospital care became equated with other basic necessities to health and well-being: food, shelter, clothing, education, medical care, and so on. Americans and Canadians living in the early twentieth century progressively subscribed to the notion that no one should be denied medically necessary hospital care for lack of means. This new, universal appeal of hospital care also brought paying patients into the hospital interior. Fees quickly became the principal income for acute-care hospitals in the closing decade of the nineteenth century, and cultivating paying clients emerged as the single most important source of institutional survival and aggrandizement.

The rapidly growing hospital establishments of North America were thus indebted to an amalgam of precepts, some ancient and others distinctively modern. There were still the venerable maxims predating the commercialization of hospital finance that defined hospitals as religious or humanitarian institutions devoted to poor relief. Hospital authorities remained wedded to the idea that hospital endeavors were still charitable enterprises and, as such, deserving of the donated time, efforts, and subscriptions of philanthropic individuals and associations. Added to these time-honored conceptions were new assumptions arising out of the secularization of hospital management, the rationalization of hospital-based professions, and the growing identification of hospital practices with scientific knowledge. Integral to these changes was the attendant notion that hospitals had the right to demand and receive fees to cover their operating expenses. Among the competing logics of the new model hospitals, at once charities for the poor and businesslike concerns for the working, middle, and upper classes, the latter surpassed the former (Agnew 1974; Stevens 1989).

This transition crowned private charitable corporations as the dominant institutions in the emerging hospital industries of the United States and Canada. Denominational rivalries among Protestants and Catholics created a permissive social context for the proliferation of private hospital charities in North America. As William Glaser has observed, in societies where one denomination clearly predominates, the church tends to surrender ownership of hospitals to government since religious leaders trust that the secular authorities will infuse hospital practices with a civic morality consistent with church doctrine (1970, 15–86). Secular management correspondingly allows religious authorities to devote more of their limited energies to propagating faith. By contrast, among those societies encompassing rival Protestant and Catholic denominations of considerable influence, owning and managing hospital charities more often becomes an extension of church efforts to attract new followers and to reaffirm the religious loyalties of current members. In each country, Protestant and Catholic populations in the nineteenth century surpassed the critical threshold required to ignite competition within the charitable establishment. Private hospitals alloyed with confessional identities predominated in North America as hospital charities made their conversion from poor relief agencies to commercial enterprises.

How do charities for the poor become institutions tinged with the aura of social prejudice and class privilege? The direct answer is that the common law not only permitted, but inadvertently encouraged, exclusionary practices. U.S. and Canadian charities derived their juridical status from the British common law of trusts. The test of charitable objects—the legal doctrine differentiating charitable from business corporations—created elastic standards for classifying hospitals as charitable institutions. The qualification of public benefit applied to hospitals stipulated that only some, not all, members of a community need derive some welfare from hospital activities for institutions to preserve their charitable status. Further, the test of charitable objects did not require hospitals to demonstrate that the poor were the exclusive, or even primary, beneficiaries of their care. The relaxed standard only required hospital charities to demonstrate that the poor were not of necessity excluded from their services. Hospitals implicitly or explicitly practicing ethnic, racial, linguistic, religious, and class discrimination did not risk losing their status as charitable institutions so long as they operated on a nonprofit basis. As far as the common law mattered, hospital charities in the United States and Canada were free to subscribe to the narrow spirit of class and ethnic feeling to raise their institutional status.

Government hospitals formed the minority among acute-care institutions for the sick in North America. The implications for the subsequent evolution of hospital policy in the twentieth century merit some elaboration. Historically, the ideological barriers to universal hospital insurance have proven considerably weaker in those nations where government authorities directly managed most hospitals. The transcendent principle of civic equality embedded in modern democratic states lends itself to making rights of citizenship the overriding consideration in hospital policy. By contrast, polities that assigned primary responsibility for hospital development to private charities commonly exhibit a different kind of political rationality. These countries risk substantial resistance to the expansion of government authority required to make hospital insurance a corollary of citizenship. Private hospitals will more likely emulate the prevailing social and economic inequalities of their surrounding societies and, thus, will inspire a climate of political opinion hostile to social leveling as made explicit in policies establishing equal access to hospital care.

Why did Canada make the transition to national hospital insurance in the postwar era while the United States did not? The answer lies in the historical emergence of publicly financed hospital care. Responsibilities for poor relief were not exclusively lodged with private charities in the time before hospitals broke free of their identification with the destitute. U.S. and Canadian governments shared these burdens with voluntary charities. But as private hospital charities manifested their commercial bias, the financial liabilities of arranging hospital care for the poor became more exclusively a governmental obligation in both countries. Tax-supported hospital care mediated the commercial transformation of hospital ventures. In each country, the turn of the century saw the emergence of public policies specifically concerned with the ends and means of government-sponsored hospital care. This first generation of hospital policy greatly differed from one country to the other and impressed very different patterns on national hospital reforms in the postwar era.

The Political Origins and Transformation of Hospital Policy

Hospital policies originated and underwent substantial revision in four distinct eras in the United States and Canada. What separated the evolution of U.S. and Canadian hospital charities from the very beginning was not the common law but constitutional and statutory laws. They assigned differing statuses to hospitals upon their inception as poor relief agencies in the first two periods spanning the late eighteenth and nineteenth centuries. In a third era, the commercial transformation of hospital finance worked in concert with political forces to differentiate statutory provisions for tax-supported hospital care from the more general trends in legislation governing public and private charity. Political reforms of the late nineteenth and early twentieth centuries not only reaffirmed important historical precedents in each country, they also codified and routinized the meanings and practices of government-funded hospital care. Federal interventions into hospital policy marked the opening of the fourth era. National policies reshaped the programmatic contours of publicly financed hospital benefits in the postwar era. Federal legislators nevertheless used the principles embedded in prewar hospital policy as the ideological templates for national reform.

The Making of Public and Private Charity in the Antebellum Era

The first two periods spanned from colonial times to the advent of confederation in Canada as it coincided with the end of the American Civil War. In these intervals the constitutional and statutory frameworks governing public and private charity gained some measure of precision in both countries. The first era witnessed the initial formation of poor relief establishments in the North American colonies. It came to a close with the onset of exceptionally heavy emigration to U.S. and Canadian shores in the 1840s. The hallmark of this first era was the uninterrupted reign of colonial approaches to financing and managing poor relief. The second era commenced with the European famines and political upheavals that precipitated large-scale Irish and German emigration to the New World and concluded with the declaration of hostilities between North and South. The defining aspect of this period was that the influx of European refugees provided a catalyst for solidifying the existing foundations of poor relief in each country. What differentiated this second era from the first was that the renewal of the U.S. and Canadian charitable establishments was accomplished under new auspices. Political parties, not colonial governors, presided over the rejuvenation of public and private charity at mid-century.

The antebellum era yielded an elementary definition of the spheres of competence assigned to public and private organizations engaged in poor relief and, further, specified their relation to one another, however crudely. These early periods bore witness to the historically contingent origins of hospital policy in the United States and Canada. In political circles there was little evidence of long-range thinking specifically devoted to the future place of voluntary hospitals in the architecture of poor relief in either country. Hospitals had not attained any sense of collective awareness or otherwise joined together to form associations for articulating political demands. To the imagination of legislators, hospital charities simply complemented much broader relief efforts and were only slightly distinguished from other benevolent societies. There was little advance warning of the dramatic transformation and proliferation of hospitals that so strikingly characterized the postbellum era. The legalities of hospital charity were correspondingly undifferentiated from, or subsumed under, broadly focused laws governing public and private poor relief. The general practices and meanings attached to public and private charity provided a few of the raw materials with which U.S. and Canadian legislators set out to construct policies uniquely bearing on publicly financed hospital care in the late nineteenth and early twentieth centuries.

Canada. Colonial legacies had a profound and lasting influence over the evolution of public and private charity in Canada. The Crown absented municipal self-government from the constitutions of Upper and Lower Canada (1791–1841), the provinces that later formed the nucleus of the Canadian Confederation of 1867. Secular authority over poor relief correspondingly fell to the provincial governments. Tax-supported charity in the nineteenth century would not develop under the direct management of local governments as typified British and U.S. practice. Of equal importance were the constitutional underpinnings of confessional dualism in Canada. The imperial government partitioned the colony of Canada into two jurisdictions according to linguistic divisions. French Catholics predominated in Lower Canada. English Protestants predominated in Upper Canada. The Crown sanctioned the consolidation of two major ethnic blocs in Canada and set in motion confessional rivalries within the charitable establishment. The emerging division of labor among the secular and ecclesiastical authorities had the Protestant and Catholic churches administering poor relief in the localities, while the provincial governments became the chief benefactors of confessional charities. From the very beginning, Canadian poor relief represented a marriage of public spending and private initiative.

The triumph of party politics militated against a complete separation of church and state owing to the unique circumstances surrounding Canadian decolonization. The winning of democratic self-government in the 1840s coincided with the fusion of Upper Canada and Lower Canada into the United Province of Canada (1841–67). The unification of French Catholics and English Protestants into a single polity, with each group enjoying evenly matched legislative representation, muted the anticlerical sentiments of democratic reformers. English and French Canadians were bent on defending and advancing their own cultural and philanthropic institutions. Canadian political parties could not subsequently forge a consensus on a secular poor relief establishment unalloyed with denominational charities. Legislators consequently spared Canada's reforming municipal governments of any mandatory responsibilities for poor relief until the late nineteenth century. Charitable institutions were left to develop under confessional auspices with continuous provincial subsidies. The prolonged synthesis of secular and ecclesiastical poor relief prevented Canadian hospital charities from assuming the legal stature of private corporations, unlike voluntary hospitals in the United States. As long as hospital charities relieved the poor on behalf of the government and received extensive provincial funding for doing so, Canadian statutes looked upon them as semiprivate, semipublic corporations.

United States. The U.S. colonial legacy represented a dramatic inversion of the Canadian experience. The Crown transmitted the Elizabethan Poor Laws to the American colonies, loading upon municipal governments direct responsibility for financing and administering public charity. State legislatures, acting as independent sovereigns in the new republic, reproduced the very image and transcript of British poor relief in the early nineteenth century. In particular, the shifting emphasis from outdoor relief to indoor relief in Britain found close parallels in the United States. Local governments progressively abandoned cash assistance in favor of investing in poorhouses. Poorhouse infirmaries became the primary loci of institutional care of the sick in the antebellum era. The secular conventions of poor relief were not the only elements differentiating U.S. and Canadian charitable establishments. The scope of confessionally inspired philanthropy also varied. Whereas Canada harbored significant Protestant and Catholic populations in the colonial era, dissident Protestant sects predominated in America from colonial times through the first half of the nineteenth century. Sectarian rivalries among Protestant churches in the United States did not exhibit the same dynamics as denominational rivalries between Protestants and Catholics in Canada. More specifically, private philanthropy in America was heavily biased toward proselytism before the Civil War. In principle, charity is a religious virtue that compels the faithful to secure their neighbors from both bodily and spiritual suffering. Material poor relief—the provision of food, clothing, shelter, and nursing care—was not the ranking concern of American religionists. As state governments did away with the last vestiges of ecclesiastical participation in secular poor relief after the War of Independence, they ceded the realm of moral causes to the churches. This left to private charities a nearly exclusive preoccupation with evangelical ministries. Unlike in Canada, the division of the labor within the American charitable establishment was not that of public financing and private administration of poor relief. Public charity catered to the body, private charity to the soul.

The apogee of party government and patronage politics in the mid–nineteenth century consolidated and intensified the divisions between secular and confessional charities. The same immigration crisis that sparked the growth of poor relief institutions under church management in Canada had the opposite effect in the United States. The municipalities shored up the secular foundations of poor relief with new investments in poorhouses and poorhouse infirmaries. Local governments would later enter the postbellum era with substantial endowments in quasi-hospital facilities. Private charities concerned with poor relief had come to perfect their specific talents as well: moral counseling of the poor; proselytizing immigrants; and exhorting the secular authorities to accelerate their efforts to substitute confinement in poorhouses for outdoor relief. The reigning orthodoxy of U.S. philanthropy at midcentury—that public and private charities operate as functionally differentiated, noncompetitive, and self-governing complements to one another—gathered additional force with amendments to state constitutions. There was some residual intermingling of public and private charity carried over from colonial times, namely, legislative supremacy over grants of incorporation to charitable institutions. However, this disappeared with the emergence of political coalitions determined to rid state governments of their legislative powers to subsidize business companies and to regulate their incorporation. The successes of the divestiture movement were embodied in new clauses of state constitutions prohibiting the mingling of public and private enterprises. These provisos vitiated state supervision over the incorporation of private charities and outlawed private charities' claims to state-legislated subsidies. In legal principle, if not always in working practice, constitutional law cemented the division of labor within the charitable establishment. Private charities would henceforth operate without any government review of their objectives and achievements apart from the juridical doctrines of the common law. Confessional charity represented an exercise in private initiative quite apart from the public interest.

Even as the purposes and practices of U.S. philanthropy achieved a remarkable degree of coherence at midcentury, there were portents of change on the horizon, many of them as yet indiscernible. U.S. charity, public and private, had given expression to the hegemony of a Protestant civic morality at the very moment that substantial Catholic minorities arrived from Europe. The addition of Catholicism to the religious mosaic did not immediately challenge the prevailing ethos of the poor relief establishment. However, Catholic doctrines and undertakings would eventually alter the course of U.S. charity in the postbellum era. The settling of Catholic immigrants into stable communities, the attendant proliferation of Catholic benevolent associations, and the growing importance of the Catholic political franchise, especially in the cities, impressed new social and political dynamics upon U.S. philanthropy. Catholicism attached great importance to relieving poverty and propagating faith as religious obligations, whereas Protestant doctrines of salvation stressed the latter. The formation of Catholic charities violated Protestant understandings of private benevolence. This breaking with convention drew Protestants into the realm of material relief in order to level the playing field of denominational competition for religious followers. This had great consequences for the subsequent evolution of U.S. hospital enterprises. The presence of a significant Catholic minority among the Protestant majority engendered the confessional rivalries necessary for the making of a hospital industry under mostly private management. Social conditions prior to the mid–nineteenth century had prefigured the emergence of a hospital industry under municipal ownership. Catholic emigration to the United States reconfigured the predestination of hospital development in a Protestant society.

The Making and Meaning of Hospital Policy

The third era coincided with the unparalleled growth of confessionally based hospital charities in the United States and Canada, beginning with the capitulation of the Southern Confederacy and ending with the onset of the Great Depression. In this period hospital policy gradually formed a distinct branch of public deliberation and action. In each country, commercialization differentiated hospitals from other charities. The other regiments of the private charitable establishment that had drawn their inspiration from benevolence toward the poor, but remained solely committed to the well-being of the unfortunate, normally experienced one of two fates. Some divisions were directly absorbed into the swelling ranks of public welfare administration in the early twentieth century. Others became dependent on public financing to the extent that their very existence hinged upon government favor. In stark contrast, an emerging partnership with the medical profession allowed private hospitals to establish a revenue base apart from the public fisc. The absorption of the hospitals into the fee-based economy of medical practice engendered a new mix of ideas and customs unique to hospital charity.

This third era saw the creation of a first generation of policies specifically confronting the problems of adjustment stemming from the commercialization of hospital finance. Policy making conformed to identical scripts in the United States and Canada. In the first instance, the aims of hospital policy became objects of explicit clarification and theorizing among legislators and private lobbies. Early phases of public deliberation exhibited shades of uncertainty about the appropriate avenues for government spending on hospital care. This ambiguity created a permissive context for experimenting with different ways of raising and distributing taxes earmarked for hospital purposes. In the second instance, legislators in each country resorted to historical precedent to surmount the controversies implied in competing policy alternatives. U.S. and Canadian governments settled the hospital question by reinstating antebellum methods for underwriting public and private charity. The irony was that legislators progressively set aside these same benchmarks in reforming policies governing other charities still devoted to poor relief. This selective restoration of antiquated charity policy carried with it the ex post facto attribution of rationality to historical practice. Antecedent policy became perceived as the natural, inevitable, and superior approach to managing the public interest in hospital care rather than a by-product of anachronistic forces.

These normalized conceptions of hospital policy owed some of their influence to the historical relationship between public and private charity, but they also borrowed much of their prestige from the reconstruction of policy making in the late nineteenth and early twentieth centuries. The inauguration of hospital policy coincided with the rise of political movements bent on remaking the legal and administrative frameworks for budgeting public expenditures. Reformers wanted politically disinterested, uniform criteria for raising taxes and allocating government spending in order to narrow the influence of political parties and to do away with the favoritism and caprice ensconced in patronage politics. Government reforms in the late nineteenth century also sought to level the inconsistencies in public policy that had long accumulated under party control over legislative offices. To the extent that administrative betterment achieved a measure of popularity, legislators identified policy making with the diminution of political patronage to mobilize latent consent for, and dissipate manifest opposition to, new policies. Hospital policy capitalized on this novel source of legitimacy. Reform legislators endeavored to formulate clearly defined regulations and standardized procedures for allocating public expenditures on hospital care. In sum, the means of executing hospital policy were employed in the service of dignifying its very ends.

The codification of hospital policy brought forward significant departures in procedure but also in philosophy. Conscious efforts to arrive at comprehensive and well-articulated statements about publicly financed hospital care engendered a gradual and unanticipated metamorphosis of the meanings attached to public and private responsibilities for hospital services. As the previous discussion suggests, tax-supported hospital charity represented a synthesis of three corresponding logics: political antiquity, political reform, and hospital reform. Integral to this amalgam were the metaphysics of the division of labor among the public and private delegations to the charitable establishments of the antebellum era. The other political ingredient thrown into the mix was postbellum government reform—the rationalization of policy making and policy implementation. In addition, there were new assumptions about hospital care stemming from the rapid proliferation of private hospitals and the advancing integration of middle and upper classes into the hospital economy. By the beginning of World War I, U.S. and Canadian laws institutionalized a new matrix of practices and meanings among the specific realms of publicly funded hospital care and the larger domains of hospital enterprising.

Canada. In the early and mid–nineteenth century, the provinces authorized subsidies to hospital charities in accordance with a number of political priorities: moderating the fiscal troubles of municipalities undergoing a painful transition to self-government; affirming ecclesiastic control over various branches of the charitable establishment; and making available enough resources to manage extraordinary demand for poor relief occasioned by peak immigrant traffic. Yet in the closing decades of the nineteenth century, immigrant claims to hospital care had declined precipitously. The settled poor were overtaking the itinerant poor as the recipients of hospital charity. The self-supporting classes increasingly patronized hospitals as fee-paying patients. Moreover, secular tendencies in provincial politics were much more pronounced, and local finances had matured to the point where the municipalities could no longer remain exempt from any obligations for poor relief. These events presented Canadian legislators with a timely opportunity to abolish public subsidies to confessionally based hospitals and establish government hospitals under municipal auspices. To the contrary, the provinces reformed antebellum methods for raising and allocating subsidies to voluntary hospitals.

The rationalization of hospital policy extended the provinces' historical role as the principal benefactor of hospital charity. Legislators retrofitted public subsidies with refinements and amendments consistent with ongoing changes in the hospital economy and with new expectations surrounding accountability for government expenditures. These regulations were given careful expression in the assorted Charity Aid Acts. This genre of legislation specifically recognized private charities as the managing partners of hospital care, standardized in exacting terms provincial obligations to supply the hospitals with working capital, and made definitive allowances for governmental oversight. The provinces subsequently passed uniform legislation mandating subsidies to publicly recognized hospitals from local governments.

This codification of the hospital subsidy laws produced a modified account of the aims of hospital policy. The provinces came to acknowledge public funding as an instrument for achieving universal access to hospital care. Provincial legislation obliged the hospitals, in spirit and in law, to admit patients on the basis of medical need while establishing an entitlement to government reimbursement for uncompensated care. The subsidy laws emerged before, and apart from, means-tested welfare regimes in the early twentieth century. As a result, hospital charity never became uniquely identified with public assistance. Municipal authorities were instructed to apply lenient standards of financial need in determining payments to hospitals for the expenses of nonpaying and part-paying patients. The cumulative effect of these reforms was to forge a single-tier hospital system. Voluntary and municipal institutions both carried the legal designation *public hospital*, meaning open to all without respect to social or economic status. Maintaining the public hospital system would later prove to be the ultimate motive of national hospital reform in the postwar era.

United States. In antebellum times the work of voluntary hospitals was largely supplementary, even if thought of as an indispensable adjunct, to the care of the afflicted in the sickness wards of municipal poorhouses and in poorhouse infirmaries. The local authorities provided for the great majority of the ailing poor. Private hospital charities employed their discretion to experiment with new educational, therapeutic, and humanitarian services. The postbellum era witnessed a dramatic reversal of fortunes of government and voluntary provisions for the sick. The social, economic, and technological changes that so strikingly contributed to the modern hospital movement made private ownership and financing the dominant forces in the U.S. hospital industry. Publicly sponsored hospital care became an adjunct to the various branches of the private hospital establishment. At the turn of the century, U.S. thinking about public and private responsibilities for hospital care underwent a transformation as had happened in Canada.

Earlier crusades against state subsidies to private enterprises had established clear boundaries between private and public charities. However, constitutional restrictions on state legislation were not generally binding on municipal initiatives. Local governments were free to employ their political ingenuity in the service of contriving precise, workable mechanisms for divorcing municipal charity from private charity or, otherwise, for marrying the two. In the late nineteenth century the great expansion of voluntary hospitals created ostensibly favorable circumstances for unifying public and private interests in hospital care. The municipal authorities had an opportunity to relinquish their troublesome investments in poorhouse infirmaries and to convert these expenses into subsidies to private hospitals. To the contrary, urban reformers were committed to building and endowing freestanding municipal hospitals for the poor in order to restore the antebellum segregation of public from private charity.

Local sovereignty over hospital policy differentiated in exacting terms the vocations of public and private institutions. Municipal ownership was perceived as an instrument for diluting partisan influences over government spending on hospital care. Hospitals under the direct management of local authorities was held out as the most promising avenue of administrative reorganization. Progressive reformers abolished, or scaled back, public subsidies to private hospitals in the cities. The courts voided public regulation of unassisted private hospitals. Public and private hospitals should not only be self-supporting, went the prescription, but also self-governing. City reformers advertised this course of action as the most logical and scientific standard for local policy. As the historically contingent origins of hospital policy became shrouded with notions of rationality, there came explicit recognition that public and private institutions occupied different ranks in a stratified hospital system. The public hospitals afforded a minimum of care to the poverty-stricken with the least interference in the affairs of private hospitals. The private hospitals carried on in the expanse above this basic level with a clear view of the commercial vistas attending the overlap of medical and hospital care. This conception of hospital care—distinctively public accommodations for the poor and separate, private arrangements for the self-supporting—underpinned U.S. hospital policy throughout the twentieth century.

The Remaking of Hospital Policy in the Postwar Era

The fourth era produced a renaissance of hospital policy beginning with the Great Depression. This period ended with the passage of capstone federal legislation that defined the scale and scope of tax-supported health insurance. This second generation of hospital policy remains the most important referent of contemporary health insurance in the United States and Canada. Policy making in this era mimicked the evolution of antecedent hospital policy. In each country the reinstatement of publicly financed hospital benefits represented an amalgam of political rationalities, historical and modern, as they combined with the logic of the changing hospital economy. Public deliberations revolved around negotiating a settlement respecting the second great transformation of hospital commerce: the acknowledged necessity of establishing insurance-based reimbursement to stabilize and enhance hospital revenues. The principal task of policy making was to adapt the fiscal and administrative contours of government-sponsored hospital care to the urgency of creating an enduring foundation for hospital insurance. The element of political modernization was that federal governments became points of convergence for political movements focused on reconstructing public financing and regulation of health care. National frameworks for setting policy added new dynamics to hospital reform, just as government reforms of the late nineteenth and early twentieth centuries mediated the articulation of the first generation of hospital policy.

Historical precedent supplied the motive force for overcoming political controversies attached to competing proposals for hospital reform in the postwar era. What was unique about this era was that hospitals had now formed associations for formulating and expressing political preferences, and so hospital lobbies also served as transmission belts for articulating and enforcing conventional notions of acceptable policy. The working consensus among legislators and hospital associations held in favor of untried methods as long as new laws remained faithful to the philosophies underlying public and private responsibilities for hospital care in the prewar era. U.S. and Canadian legislators transformed the ways and means of tax-supported hospital care while reaffirming the ideological biases of antecedent hospital policy.

Canada. Canadian hospital associations entered public deliberations over health insurance with very specific intentions. They wanted to divest provincial statutes of those provisions most resembling a poor-law approach to tax-supported hospital care: municipal certification of local subsidies for the needy. While U.S. hospitals generally preferred means-tested programs, Canadian hospitals equated them with hindrances to observing their mandate to treat all patients. The hospitals wanted more comprehensive financing and had a variety of suggestions for maintaining universal access in the era of insurance-based reimbursement. It was understood that private insurance would not cover all necessary hospital procedures and services and that even minimal protection was beyond the reach of the poor, the working poor, and those with the most serious health problems. Some Canadian hospital associations favored publicly administered universal hospital insurance. Other associations preferred universal hospital insurance under nonprofit administration. And at various times, Canadian hospitals also pledged their support for split-level insurance—a mandatory plan for most citizens and optional coverage for the wealthiest classes. Nonetheless, hospital opinion converged on the notion that broad-based, compulsory hospital insurance was necessary to level economic barriers to care.

The beginnings of a national hospital policy appeared in the early 1940s when federal committees worked out the details of a nationwide system of health insurance with the interested lobbies, namely, the national associations representing doctors and hospitals. Of its own accord, the federal government had no authority to enact a contributory insurance plan for medical and hospital care. Since the Canadian constitution gave to the provinces jurisdiction over health policy, provincial premiers held a collective veto over any federal initiative. In 1945, Canada's most populous provinces, Ontario and Quebec, refused the federal scheme because it was combined with a much more controversial proposal for redrawing the boundaries of federal and provincial prerogative over fiscal policy. In response to this first setback, Ottawa cleared away many of the hurdles to provincial endorsement of national hospital insurance. In the 1950s, the Canadian prime minister offered to move forward with national legislation with the consent of a majority of provincial governments. This promise obviated the need for provincial unanimity on health reform and, thus, greatly improved the prospects for a breakthrough. And further, federal-provincial deliberations over hospital insurance would no longer be held hostage to a consensus on fiscal policy.

In the mid-1950s, the requisite majority came from a curious alliance of the smaller western provinces and the influential Province of Ontario. The western provinces had instituted mandatory hospital insurance without federal assistance. Ontario demonstrated the most success with private insurance of those provinces bent on testing the limits of employment-based coverage. What united these provinces was their willingness to postpone deliberations over medical insurance so as to make progress on hospital reform. Setting aside this source of political controversy allowed these provinces to concentrate their energies on discovering a modus operandi for renewing their commitments to universal hospital care. With the appearance of a provincial coalition seeking grants-in-aid of tax-supported hospital insurance, the federal government was now faced with devising a national standard for the provincial hospital plans. From the standpoint of Ottawa, the government plans had several virtues: simplifying the task of engineering federal contributions, maximizing public accountability, and demonstrating the greatest potential for comprehensive and universal coverage. Ontario's willingness to accede to federal specifications would bring the entire country across the threshold to universal hospital insurance in the late 1950s. A decade later, universal medical insurance would duplicate the principles and practices of the national hospital insurance program.

United States. U.S. hospital associations entered the debate over national health insurance on very different terms from Canada. U.S. hospitals refused to ally with sponsors of progressive legislation, defined their interests against extending government sovereignty over hospital financing, and placed their hopes for reinvigorating the pay-patient trade on the expansion of nonprofit and commercial insurance. Voluntary hospitals wanted no change in the historical balance of public and private authority over hospital endeavors. The hospital associations called for strict adherence to preexisting norms of strictly controlled, but adequate, public funding for the poor and private, unsupervised financing for the working population. The Blue Cross movement opened up new possibilities for employment-based hospital insurance and was expressly launched as a bulwark against public hospital insurance. Ultimately, the pressing issue of national policy was how to assist those exiled from the private economy of hospital insurance.

Congress unwittingly eroded the infrastructure of publicly sponsored hospital care in the localities even as they knowingly dismissed any comprehensive plan for hospital insurance. Federal subsidies for hospital construction enacted in the late 1940s contributed to the relative decline of the public hospital system in the 1950s and 1960s. From the New Deal forward, federal grants-in-aid of public assistance programs also retarded the formation of adequate arrangements for purchasing hospital care for public dependents from private institutions. The exclusion of the aged and the poor from group insurance worked in concert with these other factors to create a vacuum in hospital finance. This prompted the federal government to take the lead in reconstructing tax-supported hospital care. The architecture of the Social Security Act gave federal legislators a clearly bounded response to the plight of the aged and the poor. Medicare and Medicaid programs institutionalized publicly financed hospital insurance for these groups. Where these programs strayed from precedent was to make private hospitals beneficiaries of government funding, as against the earlier convention of devoting public spending to government-owned hospitals. Though reinventing the means of providing for the dependent population, Medicare and Medicaid observed the precepts governing U.S. hospital policy from the beginning of the twentieth century. Governments would not exercise any authority over hospital affairs apart from that needed to secure treatment for the poor.

The following chapters elaborate upon the historical development of hospital policy sketched here. They illustrate a framework for understanding policy making that underscores the surpassing importance of institutional influences upon politics and lawmaking. In each country, policy innovations bearing generally or specifically on hospital care represented a confluence of three institutional forces. First, key policy changes coincided with broad-based political reforms. As Americans and Canadians reconstructed the constitutional, procedural, fiscal, and administrative bases of policy making, they created generalized opportunities for remaking policies of all stripes, not just hospital policies. Beginning with colonial forms of government, both societies reconfigured their political institutions in three major streams: democratization in the antebellum era; the postbellum reaction against legislative partisanship that sought to rationalize policy making by enlarging the scope of executive prerogative; and finally, the reconstitution of federalism inspired by the Great Depression and World War II. Each of these epochs engendered significant amendments to public regulation of hospital corporations. Second, policy reforms coincided with, and accelerated, far-reaching social and economic transformations of hospital endeavors: the commercial and therapeutic revolutions of the late nineteenth and early twentieth centuries and the second transformation of hospital finance in the mid–twentieth century.

Third, culture was the medium bridging antecedent and emergent policy. Policy making constituted a paradox. Even as legislators and lobbies sought to modernize publicly financed hospital benefits in response to political, economic, and social changes, the underlying thrusts of policy making were essentially conservative. Remaking hospital policy entailed uncertainty, controversy, and experimentation. In each country, political discord was put to rest by rediscovering and invoking the guiding principles of the preexisting legal order and then by restoring them in a new matrix of rules, regulations, and practices. Each wave of hospital policy engendered a novel synthesis of historical beliefs and of contemporary norms for realizing them.

CHAPTER 2

From Many, One: Canada's Public Hospital System

In the prewar era, government responsibility for guaranteeing universal access to hospital care became the singular integrative principle of Canadian hospital policy. This paradigm emerged out of the institutionalization of Canadian poor relief in the nineteenth century and was first articulated and codified in the Province of Ontario (Ontario 1874, c. 223). There, the provincial government had fallen into the habit of subsidizing voluntary charities affiliated with Canada's Protestant and Catholic churches to manage demands for poor relief stemming from colonization in the early nineteenth century and, subsequently, from the waves of itinerant immigrants that swept through Canada at midcentury. As the Ontario government endeavored to routinize provincial funding of voluntary hospitals in the late nineteenth century, hospital charities began to make the transition from undifferentiated poor relief agencies to centers of therapeutic nursing and medicine. The coincidence of hospital reform with political reform engendered a new synthesis of meanings and practices accorded to publicly financed hospital care. Government subsidies were no longer understood as mere instruments of poor relief but as a way of ensuring universal access to the reconstituted hospitals.

The core practices of Ontario hospital regulation were remarkably straightforward and provided the model for hospital policy for most every other province in Canada. The province mandated hospitals receiving government funding to admit patients according to demonstrated medical need. This requirement made no distinction between municipal hospitals and voluntary hospitals. Both were legally designated as public hospitals. In requiring open admissions, provincial legislation entitled public hospitals to per-diem reimbursements for hospital stays from the provincial treasury and, additionally, from local governments (Ontario 1914, c. 300). Compulsory financing of all provincially recognized hospitals became the standard for hospital legislation throughout Canada. Even though Ontario hospital policy arose out of the unique historical experience of this one province, the other provincial governments constructed the law as a rational approach to managing publicly sponsored hospital care and subsequently adopted it as the basic framework for their own hospital policies. To the west, Ontario hospital law provided the initial model for the provinces entering Canadian confederation between 1870 and 1906—Manitoba (1913, c. 28), British Columbia (1911, c. 102), Saskatchewan (1909, c. 102), and Alberta (1922, c. 60). To the east, Ontario hospital policy diffused among the older, settled provinces of the Dominion, however refractory their other political customs proved to be. It infiltrated the poor laws of New Brunswick (1917, c. 38) and Nova Scotia (1900, c. 47) and guided Quebec (1925, c. 189) as that province sought to normalize church-state relations in the provision of hospital care.

The evolution of publicly funded hospital care paralleled the rise and fall of Canada's first two constitutions and the creation of an enduring constitutional settlement attending the Confederation of 1867. In the first period, the Canadian charitable establishment emerged under the legal order erected at the convenience of the Crown (1791–1841). These arrangements set three precedents in the realm of poor relief that would later inform the elaboration of hospital policy. First, the colonial constitutions of Upper and Lower Canada—the provinces of Ontario and Quebec of present-day Canada—affirmed provincial sovereignty over public charity. Second, these same constitutions effectively recognized two established churches in the Canadian provinces—the Roman Catholic Church and the Anglican Church—and so begat the denominational cleavages that prefigured the dominant role of voluntary charities in local poor relief. In the nineteenth century, institutional care for the sick poor developed under ecclesiastic sponsorship. Confessionally based charities remained the preeminent force in Canadian hospital industry thereafter. Third, public and private charity operated in unison. The provinces provided financing for confessional charities with grants of currency and land, and the churches were put in direct charge of assisting the poor in the localities.

The second constitutional regime (1841–67) culminated in home rule in Ontario and Quebec, now joined under the United Province of Canada. Democratization engendered three developments bearing on the financing and management of Canadian poor relief. First, provincial subsidies to confessional charities became further ensconced in the political order. Second, legislators failed to draw any legal distinction between voluntary charities and those established under the auspices of Canada's reforming municipal governments. Both were considered local, voluntary institutions and operated as undifferentiated elements of a larger provincial effort to meet the needs for poor relief arising out of immigrant traffic. Third, the formation of municipal self-government reaffirmed provincial sovereignty over the Canadian charitable establishment while affording provincial legislators a generalized framework for marshaling local financing of hospital charity in the twentieth century.

In 1867, Canada's third constitution came into force as the Crown assented to the British North America Act. The act disestablished the United Province of Canada, redivided the former colony into the provinces of Ontario and Quebec, and confederated these two provinces with New Brunswick and Nova Scotia under a national parliament—the Dominion of Canada. The Confederation carried with it two transformations of provincial government. First, the provinces began to consolidate and standardize idiosyncratic legislation accumulated under the United Province. Legislative reform implied a clarification of the public interest in hospital care so as to routinize governmental funding of hospital charity. Thus appeared the first genre of legislation explicitly acknowledging hospital policy as a distinct branch of public regulation. In this era, the notion of all local hospitals constituting elements of a public hospital system first became formalized. Second, the provincial tax base temporarily eroded relative to that of the municipalities. The provinces subsequently compelled municipal governments to fund local hospital charities to compensate for declining provincial subsidies. Hospital policy restored the defining medium of colonial poor relief—the union of public financing and voluntary charity. The provinces refashioned hospital subsidies according to modern conceptions of public accountability as the hospitals were undergoing a therapeutic and commercial transformation. As the appeal of hospital care became more universal, the term *public hospital* came to signify universal access to hospital care.

The Union of Public and Private Charity in the Pre-Confederation Era

The Colonial Inheritance

Not long after the United States had found a durable replacement for the Articles of Confederation, the British set about devising some workable framework for rule in the newest province of imperial influence in North America. Canada, otherwise known as Quebec, was the tribute that the French paid the English under the Treaty of Paris in 1763. Extending from the Gulf of St. Lawrence to the western tip of Lake Erie and joined to the eastern seaboard by Nova Scotia, Canada became the nucleus of a diminished British North America. Whereas Nova Scotia possessed a colonial charter, the few provisions made for the governance of Canada accumulated detractors as British loyalists from the United States began to resettle in a predominantly French society. The influx of American expatriates to Canada revived dim aspirations for an Anglo civilization north of the thirteen colonies. Rather than level the earthworks and fortresses of the French colonial regime in Canada and rebuild anew, the Crown opted to divide the colony into two provinces—Upper and Lower Canada. (The designations *upper* and *lower* are relative to the St. Lawrence River. Upper Canada, henceforth referred to as Ontario, was upriver. Lower Canada, henceforth referred to as Quebec, was downriver.) The law of partition, known as the Constitution Act of 1791, hived off the unpopulated western reaches of Canada to provide a tabula rasa upon which English and Protestant institutions could prosper beyond the reach of French social and political customs.

The Constitution Act had a profound and lasting influence on the development of public and private charity in Canada. It militated against the formation of a secular charitable establishment under the direct control of municipal governments as would happen in the United States. The provinces became the secular authority in poor relief. Moreover, in dividing the colony of Canada into separate jurisdictions along ethnic lines—French Catholics predominated in Quebec, and English Protestants would predominate in Ontario—the Crown institutionalized confessional dualism. Local charities would develop under auspices of Canada's two established churches. Anglican and Catholic churches supplied the brick-and-mortar foundations of local poor relief, with each heavily indebted to provincial patronage.

Public and Provincial. In the absence of any well-defined municipal system, colonial governors assumed responsibility for publicly sponsored poor relief in the Canadas. Because Britain was anxious to avoid replicating any vigorous forms of self-government that had proven explosive in the American colonies, the Canadas would have no popularly elected local officials, which had been the special horror of the British experience with New England. Appointed magistrates acting through the courts of quarter sessions discharged all functions of local government (Short and Doughty 1914, 405–15). In the same spirit, the Crown overlooked the Elizabethan Poor Law as a model for colonial poor relief (Splane 1968, 65), sparing no expense to relieve local governments of any responsibilities that might assist independent action in municipal politics. Only Nova Scotia adhered to a version of the British poor laws at the time of the American Revolution, and when the Crown partitioned the western settlements of that colony to form New Brunswick, two poor law jurisdictions arose from one. The development of poor relief in the Maritime commonwealths followed the historical evolution of almshouse relief in nineteenth-century Britain and the United States (Greenhaus 1968; Hart 1958; Casidy 1945, 392–442).

In the Canadas, the ways and means of public charity followed the broader contours of provincial administration. The provinces combined highly centralized political decision making with highly fragmented administration. Early and mid–nineteenth century transportation and communication systems were rudimentary, and the absence of capable municipalities did not relieve colonial governors of the need for precinct organization. To overcome communication barriers and unfamiliarity with local conditions, provincial authorities came to depend upon an elaborate system of local agents, proprietarian and nonproprietarian, to execute government business (Hodgetts 1955). Diminutive central staffs crowned colonial departments that parceled out the substantive work of government to a maze of franchises operating in the districts. In Ontario, the two larger departments—Crown Lands and Public Works—supervised cartels of local proprietary corporations licensed to enter into contracts in the name of the Crown. The Department of Agriculture relied exclusively upon federations of agricultural associations to fulfill its purposes. In exchange for provincial subsidies, the local societies undertook a wide array of activities, most notably collecting census information on population, land use, and crop yields. As the eyes and ears of the provincial government in the localities, the Department of Agriculture also fostered all kinds of cultural, artistic, scientific, educational, and philanthropic associations. Poor relief fell under the jurisdiction of the Bureau of Colonization and Immigration. The positioning of the bureau under the Department of Agriculture corresponded to the necessity of mating the intelligence network of the agricultural societies with any serious settlement policy. The bureau adopted expedients for securing immigrant relief consonant with the generalized system of franchising public functions out to private operatives. Colonial officers redistributed immigration taxes among voluntary charities to assist their efforts to address the needs of impoverished settlers or the itinerant poor.

Private and Local. Without any commitment to positive municipal government, Canada's churches shouldered the burdens of local poor relief. In Quebec, the Crown gave free indulgence to the Roman Catholic Church's desire to preserve charity giving at the center of its religious mission: keeping French Canadians both French and Catholic. In exchange for the ecclesiastic endorsement of British governance, the imperial parliament granted the Catholic Church preeminence among the surviving institutions of the French colonial regime. The constitution of Quebec preserved the French civil code and its open-handed recognition of the primacy of Catholic parish organization in local affairs. Before midcentury, local charities prospered under ecclesiastic guidance in Quebec. In Montreal, the center of the English presence in Quebec, Protestants established nonsectarian charities. In Ontario, charitable endeavors advanced with the settling of the English population. While Catholic orders had operated hospitals since 1639 in Quebec, Protestant sponsorship of voluntary hospitals began to flourish in the 1830s, one indication of a maturing social order in the English province.

Democratization, Immigration, and Provincial-Municipal Relations

Political rivalries between Crown-appointed executives and elected assemblies, just as they proved to be the undoing of colonial rule in the American colonies, begat political instability in the Canadas (Stewart 1986). The radicalization of the lower houses in the 1820s marked the beginning of two decades of continuous struggle for democratic government in Ontario and Quebec. The Crown took different views of English and French contributions to political unrest in the provinces. The trouble in Ontario was interpreted as a crisis of self-government. The imperial parliament reasoned that English Canadians could no longer be denied their democratic inheritance as loyal subjects. Ontario was predominantly English, Protestant, and monarchist, and could be entrusted with democratic institutions fashioned according to prevailing British standards. In Quebec, the rumblings were blithely attributed to simple ethnic distemper. The lenient settlement imposed upon the French in the capitulation of Quebec in 1759 and the extended lease granted to French colonial institutions under the Constitution of 1791 were to be abrogated.

In 1841, the Crown responded to the political turmoil in the Canadas with the Act of Union. The act voided the constitutions of Ontario and Quebec and merged the two provinces into a single polity—the United Province of Canada. The new constitution of Canada made modest allowances for shifting legislative powers to the elective assembly that were consistent with limited conceptions of democratic rule in the United Kingdom. The joining of Ontario and Quebec was also a strategy for assimilating the French. The Union promised to expose the French Canadians to Ontario institutions that had now gained a measure of self-confidence and, professing the English example, to liberate the French from the institutions and traditions that threatened to impede the anglicization of British North America. The Crown did not anticipate the Canadian response to this window of opportunity. That English Canadians would settle for nothing less than democratic self-government and that the French would seize the democratic initiative to preserve their social and cultural institutions were not within the cognizance of the imperial architects of the revised Canadian constitution.

The purposes of the Union, limited democracy and unlimited assimilation, proved unrealistic. Had Ontario put assimilation before democracy, English Canadians might have pledged allegiance to a semidemocratic regime drawing upon its authoritarian reserves to cure the French, socially and culturally. English legislators did not prosecute the assimilation policy nor allow the French question to distract them from their preoccupation with democratic government. French-Canadian delegates entered the Union on the defensive but worked to expand the legislative authority of the elected assembly and mobilized French electoral representation to guarantee cultural self-preservation (Stewart 1986). As such, the Union heightened political controversy over social and cultural issues, making the defense of religion an inescapable reality of party government. Legislators subsequently extended provincial recognition and financing of confessionally based philanthropies and charities.

The province remained sovereign over publicly sponsored poor relief in Canada and did not retreat from patronizing voluntary charities. Attempts to establish capable local governments did not progress so quickly as to make municipalities a significant force in poor relief. Moreover, successive provincial administrations failed to draw any distinction between municipal charities and voluntary charities in their conception of local government and corporate charters for private relief organizations. This was typical of Canadian legislators who applied the terms *local* and *private* synonymously. The British North America Act, for example, delegated to the provinces powers over "all matters of a local or private nature" when it set out the jurisdictions of the Dominion parliament against those of the provinces under the Confederation of 1867. Municipal charities and voluntary charities shared a common status in the growing charity establishment. The province made municipal relief efforts voluntary, not compulsory. Municipal poor relief would simply correspond to the will of the local electorate, and even if taxes buttressed municipal initiatives, public financing did not generally distinguish local government charities from voluntary ones. Provincial subsidies went to both municipal and voluntary charities, and local governments generally subsidized private relief societies. In sum, the Canadian charitable establishment continued to operate on two levels as it had before the Union. In the localities, municipal and voluntary charities directly built up poor relief organization through initiative. At the provincial level, legislators confirmed and supported local efforts, public or private, with nondiscriminate financial assistance.

Public and Provincial. Provincial responsibility for poor relief was in the throes of the immigration crisis. While the province built quarantine stations for the most socially dangerous, legislators stopped short of erecting separate institutions under direct public control for the more numerous, yet less troublesome, itinerant poor. The province did not disturb established methods of subsidizing the relief efforts of confessional charities, and so poor relief was suspended in the interstices between public and private realms and between local and provincial jurisdictions. The political balance of ethnic blocs in the assembly and the divisions that appeared, or failed to appear, within those blocs weighed against the separation of church and state in the realm of charity (Careless 1967, 204–23). In particular, French-Canadian representatives served as a counterweight to the anticlerical factions of the Union and became the motive force behind the renewal of cultural and confessional dualism in Canada.

The principle of equal representation in the Union was enshrined on a regional basis, the former division between Ontario and Quebec, now corresponding to the administrative districts of Canada West and Canada East. Working majorities in the assembly were impossible to form without the collaboration of French-Canadian delegates to the legislature. The power of French Canadians within the government was continuously employed to protect against anglicization. French political strength drew from the Canadian system of representation and the groupings within it. The solidary character of Quebec legislators amplified their representation; Quebec was internally more homogeneous than Ontario. The population was primarily French speaking and Catholic, and their deputies closed ranks around most issues. Ontario was more fragmented, religiously, between Catholics and Protestants and within the Protestant sects and, politically, between classical Tories on the right and radical libertarians on the left. Therefore, majority rule in the Union was contingent on combining the voting bloc of Quebec with assorted fragments of the politically raucous English side of the province.

The settling of education policy was the political lodestar of church-state relations. The secularist factions of English Canada pressing for the separation of church and state did not cohere well enough to rob Quebec of its civil code, nor to amend the code's explicit acknowledgment of an educational system under confessional management. The Quebec delegation preserved the Catholic Church as the underpinning of French-Canadian culture, and the charitable establishment remained under comprehensive religious sponsorship. As part of a compromise with the Ontario delegation, Quebec institutionalized a Protestant, tax-supported school system for its English minority. In Ontario, the situation was reversed. The critical mass of the English-Canadian electorate favored the separation of church and state. Secularists successfully battled for divesting Ontario of an established church through the liquidation of the Clergy Reserves—the landed endowments of the Anglican Church. Dissident sects also joined together to support the creation of a secular public education system that inculcated a Protestant civic morality. But French Canadians won government sanction for a separate, tax-supported school system for Ontario's Catholic minority. Even though government had become the predominant force in public life with more limited state recognition of religious interests, the Ontario educational establishment remained implicitly confessional in its mission and organization. The charter of the University of Toronto provided an apt metaphor for church-state relations in English Canada. The province confirmed University College—a public facility—as the examining and endowment-holding body, but the larger corporation encompassed several colleges affiliated with the Catholic Church and numerous Protestant sects. This pattern of church-state federation—with the province nurturing smaller, confessionally based social institutions—also governed relations between the province and local charities.

Private and Local. With democratization came a dramatic reconstruction of the municipal system. But the movement toward public control of local institutions and the lessening of reliance upon voluntary associations for managing public services had recognizable boundaries. Poor relief most easily represented those limits. Municipal statutes left the matter entirely to the discretion of local governments (Splane 1968, 65–79). The unwillingness to fix municipal responsibility for poor relief may have had something to do with local finance. The province may have been disinclined to press local finances and administration beyond their resources. The local machinery of taxation, budgeting, and administration was still inexperienced. Municipal bond defaults multiplied throughout the latter half of the 1850s as the result of allowing local government to borrow freely against provincial credit for the construction of municipal railways (Bourinot 1887, 59). Even an obligatory poor law would have failed to become a ranking policy in the backlogged municipal agenda. Overcoming the deficit in public infrastructure accumulated in the localities from pre-Union times was a massive enterprise: building schools; paving roads; laying out sewer systems; completing bridges, tunnels, and railways; constructing public institutions like city halls, courthouses, and jails. These essential tasks of economic and political development produced more attractive claims to the local tax base.

Legislators did not insist on municipal resolution to the problem of dependency for other, less equivocal reasons. The prevalence of foreign-born poor in the localities and the close identification of voluntary charities with the province's handling of the immigration problem did not suggest that poor relief was exclusively, or even primarily, a municipal jurisdiction. Water bounded nineteenth-century Canada with twenty-four hundred miles of open navigational channels running from the mouth of the St. Lawrence River to the head of Lake Superior. Canada's urban life concentrated in port towns and cities, as did private charities that dedicated most of their efforts to succoring friendless, enfeebled, or dying immigrants. Owing to the easy passage the Great Lakes afforded to the expansive American West, the greater part of immigrant traffic comprised itinerants heading out of country. Municipal governments were reluctant to embrace responsibility for the masses of poor who were typically foreign born, had no intentions of settling, and were released upon the localities on the authority of provincial immigration agents.

Local governments struggled to find a place in an institutional landscape dominated by voluntary associations. Although municipal governments created opportunities to correct glaring deficiencies in public administration, the province's own linkages to preexisting local interests complicated the municipal role. Proprietarian and nonproprietarian agents of the provincial government held a grip on many public works that would have naturally fallen to local government under other historical circumstances. The stated preference for enumerating municipal responsibilities in a permissive, rather than imperative, voice corresponded to provincial reservations about how fast and how far local government should expand. Canadian municipal statutes favored continuity and gradualism in the unfolding of local government. The province shied away from foisting compulsory measures on local government to avoid municipal bankruptcy and disrupting provincial administration. The United Province had responded to the immigration situation in a manner consistent with colonial practices, namely, delegating local poor relief to confessional charities. The entwining of local charity in the administrative machinery of the province unified local and provincial poor relief and, correspondingly, public and private charity. Municipal statutes invited the local governments to fill vacancies in the semiprivate, semipublic charitable establishment and seek a partnership within it. The province called upon the municipalities to exercise discretion according to local circumstances as opposed to imposing obligations on local governments across the map.

Provincial-Municipal Relations. Municipal voluntarism in the realm of poor relief would not endure. In the late nineteenth and early twentieth centuries, the provinces would eventually mandate local governments to assume fiscal and administrative responsibilities for poor relief. It is essential to consider further the properties of the Canadian municipal system relative to those of the United States. The institutions of local government created vastly different opportunities for reforming public charity in each country during the waning years of the nineteenth century. The ease with which Canadian provinces codified municipal obligations for hospital charity sharply contrasted with the bitter controversy attending state oversight of municipally sponsored hospital care in the United States. Provincial-municipal relations exhibited three defining characteristics: provincial sovereignty, nonpartisanship, and uniform legislative direction.

First, provincial sovereignty over municipal corporations was fundamental in Canada. The objects of local government in Canada were twofold: to carry out the duties imposed by the provinces, to which local authorities were ultimately answerable; and to carry out the wishes of the inhabitants of the area under their jurisdiction within the scope and to the extent permitted by law. When these purposes conflicted, the priority of the former never was called into question in Canada as it was in the United States (Crawford 1954). The American colonial experience serves as a useful benchmark for understanding municipal deference to provincial legislators in Canada. American colonies were settler communities with charter privileges. Colonial rule combined democratic self-government at the local level with semidemocratic colonial parliaments. Democratization in the United States celebrated municipal autonomy and harbored a lingering suspicion of centralized administration as it connoted undemocratic, executive rule (Bailyn 1968). Nineteenth-century political movements, especially during the period of Jacksonian democracy, romanticized local government and its freedom from central authority as democratic ideals. In Canada, democratization was not highly indebted to the architecture of local government. British North America fell under imperial influence through military conquest. The right to reestablish American forms of local self-government did not follow loyalists resettling in the new provinces. The French-speaking population abandoned by France had previously lived under government from above without mediating political institutions at the local level. Reformers did not wage the turbulent battle for democracy in the name of local self-government, nor did the localities propel the democratic movement's quest for power. The arrival of municipal self-government, the extension of the local franchise, and the broadening of municipal responsibilities were by-products of democratization, not motive forces thereof.

Second, provincial-municipal relations were not implicated in party politics. The weaving together of Canada's party system came prior to the modern municipal system. When political parties were extending their reach into Canadian society, they sought out alliances with those organized segments of the population that could deliver resources and networks of influence over to party causes. Those influential institutions were more commonly churches and other voluntary associations, not embryonic local administrations. The consolidation of electoral constituencies and of local party activism gained no assistance from the geopolitical contours of local government. Nor did the province make any conscious effort to align the cascading tiers of local government introduced under the

Union with extant electoral boundaries or local party organization. The winning of self-government predestined Canadian municipal governments to a tranquil life apart from partisan politics. Local political coalitions remained aloof from provincial party organizations. Canadian forms of municipal government weighed in favor of a managerial ethic over a political one (Anderson 1972). The nonpartisan municipal ballot and the relative isolation of municipal politicking from the party system made certain that local officialdom did not complicate provincial policy making. Correspondingly, political battles emanating from provincial capitals would not continuously disrupt municipal policy making. In the United States, by contrast, municipalities more commonly adopted partisan ballots, and state-municipal relations were tainted with political rivalries between state and local party organizations.

Third, municipal legislation was uniform in Canada. Municipal law applied generally from locality to locality, not specifically. This aspect of municipal government owed its origins to the circumstances surrounding the winning of home rule in the United Province. Legislators hurriedly assembled the framework of municipal government in 1849. Municipal law took the form of a single enactment that aligned the tiers of local government—cities, towns, villages, and counties—with exacting consistency. Population centers fell into one category or another automatically and exercised powers and obligations equal to those of any other municipal corporation in the same class. Thereafter, provincial amendments to municipal law followed in the footsteps of the original statute. The United Province, and the modern system of provincial government that descended from it, legislated for one class or all classes of municipal corporations collectively rather than singling out individual localities as targets of legislative tutelage. Modest departures from this orthodoxy occurred as exceptional circumstances demanded, but they did not alter the basic approach to municipal law. In the United States, municipal legislation more commonly took the form of idiosyncratic acts. The legal basis of local government varied from one municipality to another. The accretion of special municipal law greatly compromised state legislators' capacity for transmitting policy directives to local governments on a broad scale.

The Canadian municipal system afforded legislators with a generalized framework for mobilizing local governments to achieve provincewide objectives. Its importance to the christening of hospital policy in the era of Confederation cannot be understated. Provincial governments were on the verge of standardizing the provisions of publicly sponsored hospital care in the late nineteenth and early twentieth centuries. As legislators endeavored to rationalize hospital policy, they also sought to incorporate local financing of hospital care into municipal legislation. The institutions of local government served as the orderly medium for renewing public subsidies to hospital charities.

The Making and Meaning of Hospital Policy in the Era of Confederation

The first generation of hospital policy emerged as the constitutional underpinnings of government underwent their last transformation of the century with the creation of the federal polity in 1867. Canadian hospital policy represented a confluence of three institutional forces: hospital reform, political reform, and historical precedent. Hospital reforms made institutional care for the sick increasingly distinct from other charities in the late nineteenth century. And so, the legality of publicly sponsored hospital care became progressively distinct from the other bodies of law concerned with the management of poverty. Voluntary hospitals gradually converted to domestic uses as responsibility for immigrant poor relief was transferred from provincial governments to the newly formed Dominion government. The purposes and practices of hospital care shifted. Physicians extended their reach into most every facet of hospital routine and reshaped them according to medical protocols. Urbanization wrought new economic and social realities that generalized demand for nursing care outside the realm of the family household. Hospital services would no longer bring comfort to the most pitiable only. Paying patients began to flock to hospitals for care, revolutionizing hospital administration, financing, and treatment. The therapeutic and commercial transformation of hospitals made them more universal in their appeal, and hospitals no longer understood their institutional mission as custodial charities for sick and dying immigrants.

Hospital reform coincided with political reform. As hospital policy became a specialized branch of law, it became more uniform in its application. Provincial governments set out to reform the legislative inheritance of the pre-Confederation legal order. Legislators consolidated and standardized idiosyncratic enactments that had accumulated in the mid–nineteenth century. Provincial financing of hospital care was first institutionalized through piecemeal amendments to appropriation bills whereby legislators voted lump-sum grants to hospitals on a contingency basis without reference to any transparent standard. Hospital policy, as with all other aspects of the legal order, became routinized. Legislators obliged themselves to dispense public funding for hospital care according to well-defined and consistent intentions and according to clearly articulated and uniform practices. A second, decisive element of political reform concerned the fiscal transformation of Canadian government. This required local governments to assume mandatory responsibilities for financing and administering poor relief for the first time. The United Province of Canada possessed the jurisdictions and fiscal powers of an undivided national sovereign. Most of these powers gravitated to the Dominion and left to the provinces a comparatively minor role in public finance and legislative prerogative. Direct governance of charitable institutions and local government reconstituted under diminutive provincial governments just as the municipalities cultivated administrative and fiscal competencies surpassing those of the provinces. Customs duties constituted the majority of government revenue at this time and now belonged to the Dominion. Local governments generally monopolized property taxes. A fiscal aperture was creeping open between the Dominion and municipalities under the new dispensation. The provinces would increasingly call upon the municipal fisc to underwrite the costs of poor relief in the late nineteenth and early twentieth centuries.

Historical precedent informed the substantive intent of the first generation of Canadian hospital policy. Emergent hospital law reaffirmed the institutional hallmarks of the charitable establishment under the United Province of Canada: provincial sovereignty over publicly financed hospital care; and the integration of public and private charities into a singular, unified system of poor relief. Reform legislation drew no distinctions between government and voluntary hospitals. All came under provincial supervision and financing. The historical union between the province, local government, and confessionally based charity in the provision of poor relief would endure the transformation of hospital care. Ontario was the first province to rationalize publicly sponsored hospital care. Ontario legislation gave full expression to the new synthesis of practices and meanings ensconced in Canadian hospital policy. The province's Charity Aid Act of 1874 made a formal declaration of the reciprocal obligations binding Canadian governments to local hospitals, municipal or voluntary. The act standardized provincial grants to hospital charities. Upon subsequent amendments, the law instituted uniform, compulsory grants from local governments to provincially recognized hospitals. The net result was stable financing of charity wards in all voluntary and municipal hospitals, whichever government supplied the funding. In return, the hospitals allowed themselves to be legally designated as public institutions. The legal prefix *public* attached to Canada's hospital charities had a double significance. First, the term denoted provincial sovereignty. Canadian jurists and legislators of the nineteenth century juxtaposed *private and local* with *public and provincial.* In naming hospitals as public institutions, provincial legislation identified hospital charity as a preeminently provincial jurisdiction. It was to the provinces that the hospitals were ultimately held accountable. Second, public denoted openness. The provinces indulged the parochial interests of Canadian hospitals: religious, linguistic, ethnic, and not least among them medical. But the provinces also set limits on partisanship that were consistent with government responsibility for enforcing a social minimum. Parochialism would not prejudice access to hospital care. The hospitals would satisfy the requirements of public accountability, but preserve their capacities for innovation and for promoting the social aspirations of their diverse constituencies.

Reinventing Provincial Sovereignty: Ontario Hospital Law

Ontario's hospital policy emerged as an attempt to reform ad hoc legislative appropriations to local charities that the province inherited from the Union. Ontario hospital law arose out of a dialogue between the provincial legislature and the Board of Prisons, Asylums, and Public Charities. The board had previously inspected all institutions directly established and maintained by the United Province—most of them now transferred to the Dominion government. Rather than disband the agency, the province ordered the board to conduct regular inspections of local charities in receipt of government aid and to report upon their condition (Ontario 1874, c. 224). The board did not fail to recognize the blurred distinctions between asylums, jails, hospitals, houses of industry, houses of refuge, and orphanages. All these institutions, governmental or voluntary, suffered for housing inmates whom they were not specifically designed to assist or otherwise confine. Moreover, the province's lump-sum grants lacked any methodological relationship to the actual nature or volume of the services rendered. Though the board's chief inspector advised reconstructing publicly financed relief efforts under municipal auspices, the government dismissed this suggestion and exhorted the agency to tender recommendations for standardizing provincial funding and supervision of voluntary charities. With these new instructions, the board formulated the key provisions of the Charity Aid Act, which became the modus operandi for Canadian hospital policy until the advent of national hospital insurance in the 1950s (Ontario 1874, c. 223).

The act converted provincial subsidies to local charities from lump-sum to per-diem grants so as to establish parity between the charitable services rendered and public compensation. Hospitals received more— 20¢ per diem for all admissions—and the other charities regulated through the act, namely, houses of refuge and orphanages, received less— 5¢ and 1 1/3¢ per diem. Differential subsidies advanced the triage of patients into acute-care and chronic-care institutions and fortified the distinctions between them. To this end, the province penalized subsidies for hospitals that habitually admitted chronic cases. Inmates staying over 120 days fetched a reduced per diem, inducing hospitals to house patients requiring acute care. The province required hospitals to submit their bylaws for approval so as to promote the adoption of acceptable accounting practices, prevent fraud, and accelerate the hospitals' transition from custodial to curative institutions. Any hospital qualified for provincial subsidies insofar as it accepted the regulatory provisos attached to public funding and operated on a nonprofit basis. Nonsectarian, religious, and municipal hospitals occupied a single status under the legislation. Any hospital accepting provincial support carried the legal designation *public institution.* The law did not recognize any special status for municipal institutions, nor did it initially impose statutory obligations upon municipal governments to establish, maintain, or otherwise contribute to the operations of local hospitals.

In Ontario, as in the other provinces, the government never obliged any hospital to accept public subsidies nor to accept subsidy-related supervision in the absence of governmental assistance. In practice, voluntary hospitals embraced subsidies in all but the rarest circumstances. Before the depression, government subsidies to public hospitals varied between one-quarter and two-fifths of hospital revenues from province to province. Proprietary hospitals were disqualified, while voluntary hospitals came within the orbit of government funding. In Ontario, newer hospitals were even less likely to incorporate outside of the public hospital system since provincial subsidies favored hospitals in the first ten years of operation. The province extended additional financial assistance during those critical first years when hospitals, like any other organization, seek out decisive forms of social acceptance and legitimacy. Thus, over 90 percent of acute-care beds in Canada were located within public hospitals (table 2.1).

The public hospital system mostly consisted of voluntary hospitals. In 1939, nonprofit hospitals accounted for over 80 percent of acute-care beds

TABLE 2.1.   Public and Private Hospitals in Canada, 1934

	Public	Private	Total
Number of hospitals	456 (64)	256 (36)	712
Number of beds	36,801 (91)	3,421 (9)	40,222
Admissions	541,514 (96)	24,090 (4)	565,604
Patient days	8,715,107 (95)	406,070 (5)	9,121,177
Mean stay in days	16	17	16.1
Occupancy	65%	33%	62%

Source: Data from Canada Bureau of Statistics 1936, 1011–15.

Note: Nonfederal, short-term general, and allied specialty hospitals. Percentages are given in parentheses.

in public hospitals, with the balance divided between provincial and municipal institutions (Agnew 1940, 3). Local governments did not betray any sustained interest in assuming direct responsibility for hospital care, prairie provinces excepted. There were widespread reservations in eastern and Pacific Canada about the inefficiency that would characterize municipal hospital service. Provincial laws gave no incentives for constructing municipal hospitals in the majority of provinces, and legislators generally favored voluntary ownership. The voluntary hospitals commanded the unsalaried and semisalaried labor of doctors, nurses, and other support staff, tapped into private sources of funding, and created a sympathetic and wholesome environment for recovery, attributes that municipal hospitals were not thought to possess. Municipal hospitals appeared where voluntarism proved unable or unwilling to sustain the lead, mostly in rural areas, and they reproduced the service and income patterns of voluntary hospitals. By the 1930s, government-owned hospitals occupied a distinctly junior position with less than 20 percent of all acute-care beds.

Codifying Municipal Responsibility for Hospital Charity

The rise of municipal financing of hospital care corresponded to the shifting fortunes of provincial and local fiscal capacity and the diversification of provincial responsibilities in the field of health. In the first decades of the twentieth century, municipal proceeds trebled provincial revenues (Perry 1955, 619). Moreover, provincial outlays for health services had advanced in areas only slightly connected to acute-care hospitals, which now claimed most of their revenues from paying patients. By the 1930s, subsidies to general hospitals accounted for about one-third of provincial health expenditures. Spending on mental hospitals, tuberculosis sanatoriums, and public health measures consumed the remaining two-thirds (Grauer 1939, 75). The provinces increasingly called upon local governments to uphold public obligations to cover the expense of hospital charity.

Ontario passed the Charity Aid Act of 1874 under unusual circumstances. Upon confederation, the Dominion assumed the public debt of the United Province and paid to the provinces per-capita grants out of the abundance of customs revenues. In the first few years following the introduction of dominion allowances, Ontario was running budget surpluses. This permissive fiscal context allowed the province to give generously to local charities. But the fixed Dominion grants precipitously eroded against inflation. Thereafter, the municipal tax base surpassed that of the province. The Ontario government first responded to impending revenue shortfalls with incentives for hospitals to seek out voluntary contributions from local governments, private donors, and paying patients. The Charity Aid Act was soon amended to include formulas for lessening hospital reliance on provincial subsidies. The changes introduced a fixed maximum for grants to any one hospital and instituted a system of matching grants to induce hospitals to cultivate other sources of revenue.

Ontario hospitals compensated for diminishing provincial financing. They began to attract more paying patients. Equally important, the hospitals successfully prevailed upon local governments to donate more generously, and so the source of public financing changed without falling too sharply. In 1875, the provincial treasury contributed about 50 percent to hospital revenues. In 1889, municipal grants totaled 24 percent of hospital income compared to the 34 percent originating from the province. A decade later, after the provincial government altered the Charity Aid Act to limit the scope of public funding to nonpaying and part-paying patients, provincial and municipal subsidies stood equal at about 18 percent of hospital receipts. By 1909, municipal contributions doubled provincial grants, representing 22 percent and 11 percent of hospital income respectively. In 1912, the province consolidated the regulatory advances of the original Charities Act under the Hospitals and Charitable Institutions Act (Ontario 1914, c. 300). Ontario law now compelled municipalities to contribute to public hospitals for the support of nonpaying and part-paying patients. Thereafter, provincial contributions fell. By 1920, provincial subsidies accounted for about 6 percent of the total receipts of public hospitals, and municipal contributions held steady around 22 percent as they had throughout the first decades of the century (Ontario 1875–1930). The province, however, retained control over the terms of hospital compensation, supervision, and inspection.

Ontario municipal legislation afforded the province a uniform vehicle for mobilizing local financing of hospital projects. The 1912 hospital law illustrated well this phenomenon. Mandatory subsidies applied uniformly across all levels of local government. Cities, towns, villages, and counties carried the same liability for hospital charity. It was a fixed per-diem rate payable to any public hospital—municipal or voluntary, within or outside the municipality—and conditional upon the same residency qualifications for the beneficiary. The provincial law established minimum obligations without ruling out local adaptations to suit particular needs. The hospitals and municipalities were free to enter into more generous agreements than that specified in the law or to complement it with other local arrangements. For example, the city of Toronto and its public hospitals negotiated a subsidy agreement requiring local hospitals to refer children to the Toronto Hospital for Sick Children, unless other reasons made the transferal unwise.

The transition to municipal financing proceeded under a complex balancing of rights and obligations. Provincial supervision, however, provided the integument of the subsidy policy. The government's twofold challenge was to regulate hospital incorporation to ensure that compulsory grants would not bankrupt the local fisc and to keep local per diems high enough so that public hospitals would not neglect their responsibilities for the sick poor. Ultimately, it was the province that adjudicated municipal and hospital interests. To discourage needless duplication of hospital service, the 1912 legislation strengthened the government's hand in regulating the distribution of hospital facilities. Moreover, the province bestowed powers of eminent domain upon public hospitals. The right to take lands compensated for the limitations imposed on the proliferation of hospital charities in the localities. The law empowered designated public hospitals to grow to meet demand.

Canada's Public Hospital Systems

The evolution of Ontario legislation encapsulated the general progression of Canadian hospital policy. Provincial acts authorizing subsidies made no distinctions between nonsectarian, religious, and municipal hospitals. These statutes bound local governments to this practice without exempting municipalities that operated their own hospitals. This did not distort municipal finances for two reasons. First, provincial supervision of hospital incorporation assured that hospital capacity would neither deviate from local demand for care nor from local capacity to underwrite hospital enterprises. Second, with obligations for the poor evenly spread over the public hospital system, local government hospitals did not normally require any more tax support than voluntary hospitals. Municipal hospitals also derived the great majority of their revenues from paying patients.

Though the core elements of Canadian hospital policy were essentially similar, provincial budgets varied as did patterns of municipal involvement in hospital management. These differences produced regional diversity in hospital ownership. Where provincial funding consistently exceeded municipal subsidies or where municipal institutions were otherwise comparatively weak, voluntary sponsorship of hospital undertakings was paramount. In Quebec, provincial subsidies to public hospitals ranged from two to four times greater than municipal allowances. Combined provincial-municipal subsidies peaked at 40 percent of hospital revenue in the depression. Government funding mostly went to hospitals under the direction of Catholic nursing orders (Quebec 1914–40). In British Columbia, where provincial and municipal grants routinely comprised 40 percent of hospital income in the 1920s and 1930s, provincial funding generally accounted for 60 percent of hospital subsidies (British Columbia 1926–36). Both public hospital systems almost entirely consisted of voluntary hospitals. By the 1950s, voluntary hospitals accounted for 95 and 98 percent of bed capacity in the two provinces (table 2.2). In Prince Edward Island, municipal government was rudimentary. All of that province's hospitals developed under voluntary sponsorship. Where the province was the principal philanthropist, the donations went to voluntary hospitals. No exceptions are needed to prove the rule. Even though Ontario made local governments carry the larger burdens of publicly financed hospital care, the province held direct responsibilities for those living in unorganized territories awaiting the formation of municipal corporations. In lieu of establishing government hospitals to bring medical attention to the hinterland, the province relied on the Red Cross Society to build outpost hospitals—totaling 24 by 1928—with provincial funds.

Where responsibility for hospital subsidies came to fall more decisively on the shoulders of the municipalities, noticeable divisions occurred between the older, settled provinces of New Brunswick, Nova Scotia, and Ontario and the more recently established provinces of Alberta, Saskatchewan, and Manitoba. In the east, municipal hospitals generally arrived after the core of the hospital industry emerged under voluntary management. There, local government hospitals were the unanticipated offshoots of growing municipal responsibilities for health and welfare. With modest exceptions, these institutions tended to serve as the only vehicle for hospital care in their communities. By contrast, western Canada did not discourage municipal hospitals. Government hospitals in Alberta, Manitoba, and Saskatchewan were the primary response to shortages of facilities in rural areas. Voluntarism was a force in the west, but primarily in urban centers. The city of Winnipeg satisfied its hospital requirements entirely with Protestant and Catholic institutions, corresponding to eastern patterns. As the entrepôt for the western agricultural economies in both finance and transportation, Winnipeg fostered a comparatively advanced philanthropic class that buoyed the city's voluntary hospitals. Aside from the large Protestant hospitals in Winnipeg, Catholic nursing orders managed most voluntary hospitals in the west. By 1930, Edmonton had three Catholic hospitals, and Calgary operated two. Catholic hospitals also formed the primary complement to municipal hospitals in the more numerous, smaller cities like Saskatoon and Regina.

The western provinces called upon the most concentrated mechanism of social cooperation—the municipal system—to respond to rural hospital needs. Between 1910 and 1930, rapid settlement produced scattered rural communities with limited economic and social capital, and so voluntarism alone could not surmount the challenges of hospital construction and

TABLE 2.2. Ownership of Public Hospitals in Canada, by Province, 1957

	Public Hospitals	Beds	Provincial Hospitals (% of total beds)	Municipal Hospitals (% of total beds)	Nonsectarian Hospitals (% of total beds)	Religious Hospitals (% of total beds)
Newfoundland	38	1,701	29 (56)	—	6 (25)	3 (19)
Prince Edward Island	8	657	—	—	6 (68)	2 (32)
Nova Scotia	45	3,322	1 (17)	7 (22)	28 (31)	9 (31)
New Brunswick	34	2,461	1 (3)	5 (20)	13 (30)	15 (46)
Quebec	131	24,211	1 (1)	2 (1)	38 (32)	90 (67)
Ontario	205	29,379	—	20 (19)	138 (51)	47 (30)
Manitoba	73	4,611	—	52 (32)	8 (32)	13 (36)
Saskatchewan	150	5,984	5 (9)	119 (64)	4 (1)	22 (27)
Alberta	102	7,368	1 (14)	61 (49)	4 (3)	36 (34)
British Columbia	96	7,807	1 (3)	2 (2)	69 (68)	24 (28)
Canada	894	88,158	41 (4)	268 (18)	315 (37)	270 (41)

Source: Data from Canada Bureau of Statistics 1957, 1:42–43.

Note: Nonfederal, short-term general, and allied specialty hospitals. Canadian totals include public hospitals in Yukon and Northwest Territories. Percentages may not sum to 100 due to rounding.

management. By the 1920s, Alberta, Manitoba, and Saskatchewan passed legislation enabling the formation of union hospital districts (Alberta 1922, c. 116; Manitoba 1933, c. 15; Saskatchewan 1920, c. 213). These acts empowered towns, villages, and rural municipalities without sufficient resources to independently maintain hospitals to form special-purpose districts with adjoining municipalities. District boards levied property taxes to fund the construction and operation of union hospitals for the combining local governments. By 1937, 22 union hospitals served over one-half of Alberta's rural population (Alberta 1938, 282). By 1930, Saskatchewan had 20 union hospitals, multiplying to 78 in the 1940s (Taylor 1987, 71). Over the long run, the proliferation of these hospital districts intensified the geographical separation of municipal and voluntary hospitals in Canada. On the eve of national hospital insurance in 1957, Canada possessed 268 municipal hospitals, and the three prairie provinces housed 232 of them (table 2.2).

Conclusion

The paradigm of Canadian hospital policy had complex historical roots. The incipient supremacy of colonial governors over secular poor relief made the provinces the chief underwriters of hospital finance in the nineteenth century. The entrenchment of cultural dualism in Canada anointed confessionally based charities as the dominant force in local poor relief and as the primary beneficiaries of provincial spending on hospital care. The fusion of Ontario and Quebec into a common polity denied the secularist factions of the Union a commanding role in Canadian politics at midcentury. And so, the marriage of convenience between church and state became the enduring foundation of the Canadian charitable establishment.

Canadian municipalities, though largely inert during the nineteenth century, came to play a significant role in hospital financing at the turn of the century. Their part radically differed from that of U.S. local governments as will become evident in the following chapter. Whereas Canadian municipalities allocated hospital subsidies according to provincial design, state supervision of locally financed hospital charity remained slight and ineffective. In Canada, local spending primarily went to provincially recognized voluntary hospitals. In the United States, local governments circumvented voluntary hospitals in making arrangements for the poor in favor of erecting separate hospitals under municipal ownership and control. The dividing factors were the constitutional and legislative underpinnings of municipal rule. Canadian municipal law served as an efficient conduit for transmitting provincial objectives to local governments with a minimum of disturbance. The provinces favored voluntary management wherever possible, and when they turned to local administrations to bolster public financing of hospital care, the provinces conveyed this same preference to municipal governments.

Finally, the socioeconomic transformation of hospital endeavors changed the meaning of government subsidies. The original dispensation was geared to addressing the needs of friendless and diseased immigrants who endangered the health and well-being of the settled population. The dramatic lessening of the public health risks associated with immigration, the subsequent integration of the local poor and the self-supporting into the hospital interior, and the secularization and medicalization of hospital practices transformed the significance of public funding and regulation of hospital care. Legislators no longer identified hospital policy with the maintenance of institutions for the exclusive use of the poor but with the objective of reserving a place for all patients in the reformed hospitals. Universal access became the unifying principle of publicly sponsored hospital care in Canada.

CHAPTER 3

The Tiering of the U.S. Hospital System

Before the Great Depression, public institutions for the poor and private institutions for the self-supporting became the singular integrative principle of U.S. hospital policy. This paradigm grew out of the institutionalization of nineteenth-century poor relief. U.S. law partitioned the charitable establishment into two functionally differentiated, self-governing branches—one public and the other private. In Canada, the presiding logic of poor relief was that of synthesis. The incipient fusion of provincial, municipal, and voluntary relief efforts culminated in a public hospital system that represented a union of public financing and private provision. In the United States, the governing logic of poor relief was that of division. Beginning in colonial times and through successive reforms of state and local governments, Americans progressively segregated the financing, organization, and management of public charity from private charity. The fragmentation of poor relief prefaced the reconstruction of hospital charity in the late nineteenth century. The explosion of private hospitals drawing income from paying patients coincided with the expansion of publicly owned and financed hospitals for the poor. From the emergence of this two-tiered hospital system, U.S. legislators and voluntary hospitals derived the maxim of hospital policy. Public authorities would see no farther than the needs of the poor. Distinctive, private institutions would provide for the hospital needs of the self-supporting.

Twentieth-century hospital policy traced its origins to incipient patterns of U.S. constitutional and statutory law, the reconstruction of the U.S. government attending the democratization of the franchise in antebellum times, and the rationalization of the municipal political order during the progressive era. In the first period, American legal conventions set two important precedents in the realm of poor relief that would later inform the elaboration of hospital policy. First, colonial law affirmed municipal sovereignty over public charity. State governments reconfirmed the Elizabethan Poor Laws as the model for American poor relief in the early years of the new republic. The principle of local responsibility specifically called for the use of municipal taxes to fund poor relief, granted local governments maximum discretion in determining the amounts raised, and produced little state supervision over local relief practices. Second, state legislators excluded the ecclesiastical authorities from the management of secular poor relief. This exemption, combined with the prevalence of dissident Protestant sects in the American colonies, infused private charity with a uniquely spiritual mission. Whereas the municipalities directly assembled the material infrastructure of poor relief, confessionally based philanthropy specialized in the ideological branches of charitable endeavors: the advancement of religion and the advancement of education. Thus, American charitable establishment first exhibited a division of labor between the secular and ecclesiastical authorities. Public charity comforted the body. Private charity comforted the soul.

From the 1820s to the Civil War, democratization carried with it three developments that abetted the divisions within the U.S. charitable establishment. First, the immigration crisis dramatically enlarged public relief efforts just as local overseers were abandoning outdoor relief in favor of indoor relief. In colonial times, local overseers commonly extended poor relief in the form of cash payments, food, and medicine to the poor in their own homes. In the 1820s, local overseers increasingly relied upon the discipline of the poorhouse to deter the poor from seeking charitable assistance. Poor-law authorities also maintained separate sickness wards for the aged and the infirm in local poorhouses. In some cities, separate poor-law infirmaries appeared as part of larger poorhouse complexes. Since freestanding hospital charities were rare before the Civil War, poorhouses provided the only place of refuge for most of the sick poor. Thus, U.S. cities would later enter into the era of rapid hospital expansion with significant investments in quasi-hospital facilities. Second, revisions to state constitutions deprived state legislatures of the authority to finance and regulate private charity. The division of labor between secular and religious philanthropy was now reinforced with constitutional edicts separating the finances and management of public and private charities. And third, the legal partitioning of the charitable establishment into two self-governing branches prefigured the advancing disintegration of secular poor relief into two independently financed and regulated domains—one under state jurisdiction and the other under municipal control. As political parties extended their reach into state and municipal politics in the antebellum era, legislative oversight of local government became increasingly contentious and would eventually inspire a municipal revolt against state tutelage of local policy making.

In the progressive era, the first generation of hospital policy emerged as urban reformers endeavored to rationalize the foundations of municipal rule. The political thrusts of municipal reform—liberating urban governments from state legislative oversight, rolling back partisan influences over local policy making, enlarging the prerogative of the executive branch of government, and codifying and standardizing the ends and means of publicly sponsored hospital care—combined with the rapid expansion and commercial transformation of private hospitals to institutionalize a two-tiered hospital system. The rationalization of publicly sponsored hospital charity restored the institutional motif of antebellum philanthropy: the division of the U.S. charitable establishment into two functionally differentiated and self-governing branches. Progressive reformers envisaged municipal spending on municipally owned hospitals to the exclusion of subsidizing private charities in fulfilling local obligations to the sick poor. City governments signed into law extensive investments in public hospitals in the first decades of the twentieth century. Progressive reforms effectively differentiated public and private institutions in the emerging hospital industry. Public hospitals descended from poorhouses, derived their finances from municipal budgets, and succored the poor. Confessionally based hospitals predominated within the private hospital system. These voluntary hospitals rose to preeminence on fees from paying patients. Public arrangements for the poor and private arrangements for the self-supporting became the leitmotiv of the U.S. hospital system.

The Separation of Public and Private Charity in the Antebellum Era

The Colonial Inheritance

The legalities of the U.S. charitable establishment were derived from English statutory and common law. British precepts governing charitable undertakings had their origins in two statutes passed by the Tudor parliament in 1601: the Elizabethan Poor Law and the Statutes of Charitable Uses. Together, these acts defined the several meanings of charity and gave legislative blessing to a dual system of poor relief—one secular and public, the other ecclesiastical and private. The Elizabethan Poor Law established a statutory framework for publicly financed and administered poor relief. The Statute of Charitable Uses codified the legally permissible objects of private charity. There were three major headings enumerated in the Statute of Charitable Uses: the relief of poverty, the advancement of education, and the advancement of religion. Corporate bodies devoted to these purposes were classified as charitable institutions. They were entitled to receive bequests, donations, and fees without penalty of royal taxation. Also exempted from taxation were the corporate assets of charitable institutions. In the domain of poor relief, the Elizabethan Poor Law and the Statute of Charitable Uses failed to draw clear lines of responsibility among public and private charities. This ambiguity was a source of persistent controversy in the elaboration of the British social policy in the eighteenth, nineteenth, and early twentieth centuries.

Since the political and social landscapes of the United States and Canada were sufficiently different from that of England, the incipient frameworks of British law were modified in their applications in the North American colonies. In Canada, colonial governors claimed only one-half of their legal inheritance in the realm of poor relief—the Statutes of Charitable Uses—and overlooked the Elizabethan Poor Laws as a blueprint for secular relief. Thus, Canadians sidestepped the jurisdictional disputes between public and private charities that often haunted the United Kingdom. The resolution to the problem of counterpoising public and private charity was to meld them together into a unified relief network. In the United States, the solution to the riddle of balancing public and private charity was not found in synthesis but in division. Americans partitioned their charitable establishment into functionally differentiated branches. The settlement governing the separation of church and state vested the secular authorities with the initiative in poor relief. The ecclesiastical authorities more commonly devoted themselves to the other objects of charity: the advancement of religion and the advancement of education.

Public Charity. Secular poor relief in the American colonies recapitulated in broad outline the essentials of the Elizabethan Poor Law but with some early differences (Trattner 1984, 1–15; Rothman 1971, 3–29). In Britain, the poor laws broke with the tradition of easing the distress of the poor through voluntary subscriptions to poor relief funds. The legislation created a secular, tax-supported system, locally financed and administered. Poor relief centered on the triage of public charges into two broad categories—the impotent poor and the able-bodied poor. Impotent cases comprised the aged, the sick, and those matching any one of a rich array of descriptions for mental illness. Their care was more often institutional in places such as asylums, almshouses, or poorhouses, otherwise known as indoor relief. For the able-bodied, local governments were expected to dispense outdoor relief and couple public assistance with the threat of enforced work routines to prevent chronic dependency. Although the poor laws called for the careful differentiation of relief practices for one class of poor and the other, the dividing line passed out of vogue with the confirmation of the New Poor Laws in the 1830s. Local overseers of the poor began to congregate all public dependents within poorhouses. Consistent with British practice, American poor laws held local governments responsible for the poor settled within their boundaries. Contrary to British practice, American poor laws initially placed little emphasis on indoor relief. Outdoor relief was paramount. Colonial laws specified a continuum of provisions for various dependents, ranging from enforcing familial obligations of settlers to support their own relatives, to binding out deserted or orphaned children to apprenticeships, to contracting out the able-bodied to the lowest bidders, and to outdoor relief for the aged and sick in their homes. Only later would American and British patterns of secular poor relief converge on the poorhouse model.

Private Charity. Confessionally inspired benevolence had an overtly spiritual bias before the Civil War. The secularization of poor relief before and during the Revolution left to America's Protestant sects a nearly exclusive preoccupation with moral crusades spanning all kinds of proselytizing and educational endeavors (Bremner 1980, 14–34). Evangelism absorbed most of the energies and resources of private philanthropy. Missionary, tract, Bible, and Sunday school societies drew upon the organization and finances of dissident Protestant sects. And, sectarian rivalries also drove the proliferation of academies, colleges, and universities. Material poor relief remained largely absent among the achievements of U.S. voluntarism. To the extent that private charities devoted their efforts to ameliorating poverty, they did so in a manner consistent with the explicitly moralizing orientation of Protestant doctrine. The mission of New York City's Association for Improving the Condition of the Poor (AICP) illustrated well the selective interests of Protestant charitable establishment in poor relief. Organized in 1843, the AICP provided the model for female benevolent societies in cities and towns across the country at midcentury (Katz 1986, 58–84). The association concentrated its energies on achieving two principal aims. The first of these was political. The AICP consistently pressed local governments to abolish outdoor relief. The AICP reasoned that poverty stemmed from the moral failing of individuals. It was the association's considered opinion that cash assistance habituated the poor to a life of indolence and sapped their determination to become self-supporting. Consistent with this belief in the individual causes of poverty, the association lobbied to institutionalize workhouses and poorhouses as the primary vehicle of public charity. Forced labor within the workhouse would recondition the idle poor to a life of productive vocations as well as deterring charity abuse. Second, the association took moral counseling of the poor, not material assistance, as the primary focus of its own immediate efforts to alleviate poverty. The AICP was the forebear of the Charity Organization Societies—the coordinating bodies and political arms of the Protestant poor relief establishment—that proliferated across the country in the postbellum era.

Democratization, Immigration, and
State-Municipal Relations

In the 1820s, the democratization of the franchise carried with it rapid and sustained constitutional amendments to the procedural and substantive frameworks of legislative rule. The notion of the sovereignty of the people materialized in new laws detailing procedures for invoking constitutional conventions, popular initiatives, and referenda (Bryce 1891, 1:413–57). The constitutional underpinnings of Canadian democracy provided a stark contrast to those of the United States. In Canada, democratization required provincial legislators to subvert their colonial constitutions but to preserve them as fictional representations of the political order as part of their allegiance to the Crown. Canadian legislative conventions were primarily unwritten, developed through the party system, and consequently were not subject to amendment at the behest of the electorate. In the United States, the plebiscite emerged as the fourth branch of state government. Over the course of the nineteenth century, constitutional revisions narrowed the discretion of state legislatures in almost every detail: limitations on public debt and taxation, prohibitions on special and local acts, enlarged gubernatorial and judicial powers, and other directives liberalizing incorporation laws routinely appeared in state constitutions. By 1887, the forty-two U.S. states had collectively adopted no less than 105 distinct constitutions and 215 packages of amendment to them, some minimal, some extensive (Hitchcock 1887, 13). By the twentieth century, state constitutions were intricate documents, loaded up with many details of what would have otherwise been recognized as statutory law (Dealy 1914, 214–41). The micromanagement of legislative behavior through constitutional referenda lasted well into the twentieth century (U.S. Commission on Intergovernmental Relations 1955). These constitutional amendments effectively dismantled legislative sovereignty over the United States' public and private charitable establishments.

Constitutional law intensified the divisions between the public and private charity. Confessionally based charities became classified as private corporations under widely adopted constitutional amendments that forbade state governments from granting incorporation through legislative acts. The new procedural foundations of incorporation divorced public regulation from legal grants of corporate status. Henceforth, voluntary charities incorporated without any public supervision of where they located or what services they performed and without any reasonable expectation of government subsidies for their efforts. The introduction of general incorporation laws also came with prohibitions against state financing of private corporations and, subsequently, other legal impediments to state-legislated contributions from local governments to private enterprises. The pressures of midcentury immigration did not result in a union of forces among state governments and private charities comparable to the continuing rapprochement of provincial governments and voluntary charities in Canada. State governments generally entered the postbellum era without the legal authority to subsidize or regulate private charities and without any constitutional warrant to compel local governments to do the same. In the United States, the constitutional order precluded the formation of hospital policies akin to those of Canada, which were predicated upon compulsory provincial-municipal subsidies to voluntary hospitals.

The abolition of state sovereignty over the private philanthropy coincided with the dramatic reconstruction of the public charitable establishment. First, the immigration crisis prompted an escalation of state and local spending on poor relief. Rather than expend government finances on cash assistance to the poor as had been the norm in earlier periods, Protestant social reformers successfully rededicated public relief budgets to the construction and maintenance of poorhouses. Confining the poor to institutions made municipal almshouses the dominant loci of care for the sick poor. In this era, local governments acquired significant investments in poorhouse infirmaries. These accommodations prefigured the emergence of special-purpose municipal hospitals for the poor alongside the proliferation of voluntary hospitals after the Civil War. Second, the extension of party politics to local governments in the first half of the nineteenth century created political turbulence between state legislatures and local governments that ultimately eroded state sovereignty over municipal poor relief. The implication of municipal legislation in partisan politics created an impasse in state-municipal relations in the latter half of the nineteenth century. This stalemate eventually generated legal and political barriers to legislative oversight of local charity giving. Just as state constitutions formalized the legal separation of public and private poor relief, these same constitutions increasingly partitioned government authority over publicly financed and administered charity among state and local governments. The constitutional balance of power weighed against state prerogative and in favor of unmediated municipal self-direction in providing hospital services for the poor.

Public Charity. By midcentury, state and local overseers progressively curtailed outdoor relief—cash, food, clothing, and fuel extended to the poor in their homes—in favor of confining public dependents to institutions. Indoor relief within poorhouses moved to the forefront of public policy. Colonial settlers had normally relied upon poorhouses to isolate the wandering poor who were anomalies in a poor relief system premised upon settlement laws. In the 1820s, charity reformers reappraised the formerly limited uses of the poorhouse. They now intended to substitute almshouse care for the inhumane practices that had grown up around the contract system whereby local overseers auctioned out the poor to those willing to accept the lowest payment for assuming responsibility for public dependents. Moreover, outdoor relief to the able-bodied was now thought to weaken the moral fiber of the poor as it would destroy their resolve to become self-reliant. The reformed poorhouse would ostensibly provide comfort to those who could not care for themselves—the feeble, the aged, and the sickly—and enforce work routines for the able-bodied in order to make them contribute to their upkeep. Informed opinion anticipated a central role for the poorhouse in rehabilitating individuals and returning them to their communities as self-reliant, morally disciplined citizens (Rothman 1971, 155–79). At midcentury, the fate of the poor became nearly indistinguishable from the fate of the immigrant. Immigrant poverty robbed poorhouses of any rehabilitative pretensions as the cultural leanings of immigrants made them unlikely suspects for moral instruction. In principle, state and local governments stood behind institutionalizing the lower classes and foreign born as the preferred vehicle of public charity, but indoor relief never completely eclipsed outdoor relief (Rothman 1971, 178–205; Katz 1986, 3–34). Nonetheless, institutional charity for the sick poor overwhelmingly developed within local poorhouses in the United States (Rosenberg 1987, 18–19), whereas voluntary hospitals became the primary custodians of the immigrant sick in Canada.

Private Charity. At midcentury, voluntary charities became private corporations as plebiscites ratified constitutional prohibitions against special incorporation laws and state subsidies to private associations. Before these constitutional amendments, incorporation was a legislative privilege. Incorporation for expressly private purposes did not exist. Legislators linked corporate status to the furtherance of public purposes and balanced the social utility of corporate functions against the self-regarding motives of those petitioning for incorporation. Corporate charters were statutory instruments, and legislatures reserved the authority to amend corporate bylaws, to fix the composition of governing boards, and to advance public credit or capital for corporate purposes. The passage of general incorporation laws undermined the legal conception of corporate power as a concession of the state (Millon 1990).

Constitutional stipulations for general incorporation laws were originally formulated to safeguard the public treasury from incurring any further debts as a result of state subsidies to business corporations. In the early nineteenth century, economic growth had fueled demand for company charters that often conferred exclusive or near exclusive privileges upon successful applicants. Land companies, banks, turnpike, canal, railroad, and other public utility companies, and, last, manufacturing and trading companies resorted to the legislatures for the legal and financial privileges entailed in earlier forms of incorporation (Seavoy 1982). By midcentury, states had imprudently borrowed money to finance many of these enterprises, guaranteed the debt of many others, and consequently accumulated unprecedented public deficits. In response, constitutional referenda affirmed injunctions against incorporating businesses and charities under special acts. Legislatures could no longer pass any law that could be interpreted as conferring a grant of exclusive privilege or immunity upon any singular corporation. This transformed what were heretofore considered semipublic, semiprivate corporations into uniquely private organizations. The public interest and public finances were separated from incorporation procedures. Corporate law now made incorporation a right, and voluntary charities incorporated by filing articles of association with county clerks or judges. Before the depression, voluntary hospitals incorporated apart from any form of public regulation except in New York. That state was the only one requiring private hospital charities to obtain the approval of a supervisory board before a county official issued a certificate of incorporation (Lapp and Ketcham 1926, 49–93).

Although public funding of charitable institutions had not encouraged legislative impropriety, state governments no longer possessed the authority to enact subsidy policies comparable to those in Canada. General incorporation laws arrived with blanket prohibitions against state appropriations to private corporations. The purest separation of public finance from private charity occurred outside of New England and the Mid-Atlantic states. A 1901 survey conducted under the auspices of the National Conference of Charities and Correction spotted unimpressive examples of state subsidies to private charities outside of the Northeast. But even there, public subsidies were diminishing (Barbour et al. 1901, 119–31). The middle, western, and southern states enacted constitutional laws against the mingling of public and private enterprises that institutionalized the separation of public and private charity before their fledgling charitable establishments embarked upon extensive poor relief operations. Even though many constitutional amendments progressively rescinded prohibitions against state funding of private charities in the early twentieth century, as late as 1929, twenty-six state constitutions still forbade public appropriations to private charities. But only five constitutions expressly prohibited municipal governments from voting subsidies to private charities (Johnson 1931).

Lingering subsidies to private charities primarily generated controversy in the older states of the Northeast. And, these controversies appeared in the postbellum era. The older states had subsidized voluntary charities in the early and mid–nineteenth century, and they soon faced the prospects of voiding subsidies or exempting them from constitutional injunctions. In the antebellum era, state subsidies to private charities did not attract much scandal. Insofar as voluntary charities behaved in non-controversial ways and operated in a sphere of recognized public competence, their growth promised to lighten the burdens of state and local overseers of the poor. Northeastern states often extended timely assistance to private charities by contributing to their endowments upon incorporation or by special allowances to absorb deficits that otherwise threatened their solvency. The low volume of private benevolence implied that even irresponsible subsidies could not have depleted the state treasury on a scale approaching the losses associated with business concerns. Voluntary charities operated at the margins of municipal poor relief before the Civil War. However, the arrival of Catholic minorities ignited denominational rivalries in the private charitable establishment that greatly accelerated the founding of voluntary charities after the Civil War. Only with this unforeseen proliferation of private charities did public subsidies suffer the same kind of political attacks hurled at state aid to profit-making enterprises.

The Immigration Crisis. The overall response of New York State's charitable establishment to the immigration crisis commands attention. In the antebellum era, that state bore the brunt of European immigration to U.S. shores, and its legislature took an active hand in dispensing relief to impoverished and diseased passengers of immigrant ships. The Empire State also harbored the most ethnically diverse population in the country, which had made some elementary progress in establishing private charities for the poor: immigrant aid societies and an array of makeshift orphanages and hospitals. Because New York labored under the dilemma of immigrant poor relief as did the United Province of Canada, it offers an instructive comparison.

The state of New York had recognized a special category of poor under its charge since the Revolution. The devastation suffered in New York during the War of Independence had given rise to a class of refugees seeking assistance who did not properly fall within the jurisdiction of the localities. Hence, New York entered the nineteenth century with a state poor law that brought it into the fray of immigrant relief. Immigrant poverty had disrupted the normal execution of local poor relief as early as the 1830s but overran it in the 1840s. Local overseers reluctantly accepted immigrants into their charge, but the state evidently had a legal responsibility to assist the municipalities in their efforts to cope with them. Under pressure from local governments and immigrant aid societies, the state established a poor relief board in 1847, the Commissioners of Emigration. The commissioners maintained the state's first ever standing organization in poor relief. Empowered to inspect ships landing in New York harbors and to levy indemnities against shipmasters for passengers likely to become public charges, the commissioners soon commanded a significant share, albeit still a minority one, of poor relief funding in the state. In addition to financing and managing quarantine hospitals in the New York City harbor, the commissioners distributed over $800,000 among local charities, public and private, between 1847 and 1860 (Schneider 1938, 295–316).

The commissioners did not unify public and private charity in the state even though they brought many orphanages, hospitals, and other charities, public and private, within the orbit of state finance. Private charities were not preferred in the allocation of poor relief funds. The vast majority of the commission's disbursements, about 90 percent, landed in the accounts of city, county, and town overseers. And, the agency accepted liability for immigrants only, implying no attempt to influence the overall conduct of local poor relief. The commissioners did not create any opportunity for state officials to gain leverage over relief granted to the local and settled poor in either public or private institutions. Sporadic budgeting of subsidies to private charities reflected a willingness on the part of the commissioners to treat them as auxiliaries to, rather than integral components of, public relief efforts. And even though the commissioners more regularly patronized the poor relief administrations of the municipalities, they did not monitor local applications of state funding.

The 1850s marked the apogee of state involvement in local charities in the nineteenth century. The power of the Commissioners of Emigration declined precipitously during the Civil War when immigration dwindled, never to return to its antebellum strength. In the postbellum era, the health and welfare of landed immigrants improved greatly with new protective legislation regulating the conditions aboard immigrant ships. Further, the social mechanisms of channeling immigrants into settled lives had matured with the securing of ethnic niches in the economic, political, and social life of the nation. In the 1890s, the much diminished infrastructure of the Commissioners of Emigration passed into the hands of the federal government when Congress first assumed singular control over immigrant medical relief.

The North American immigration boom of midcentury failed to draw public and private charity closer in New York. The crisis of immigrant poverty abetted the rapid expansion of municipal poor relief. No sustained attention was paid to incorporating private charities into a unified relief effort, which was the hallmark of the Canadian charitable establishment. The immigration crises struck too early to give private charities any decisive role in alleviating increased demand for poor relief. In the antebellum era, private associations were nearing, but had not yet embarked upon, significant investments in benevolent institutions. The great proliferation of private charities extending material relief, most notably hospitals and orphanages, commenced in earnest after the conclusion of the Civil War. For the time being, material relief fell under the jurisdictions of state and local overseers while moral assistance remained within the province of private philanthropy. Further, local control over poor relief survived the immigration crisis of midcentury without substantive amendment. No enduring form of state supervision accompanied state funding of local charities, public or private. Equally important, the established method of local relief—the poorhouse—also survived the anomaly of immigrant relief and prefaced the dramatic explosion of local poor relief agencies, public and private, in the postbellum era.

The Incipient Municipal Revolt. Relations between state and local governments became increasingly contentious in the mid–nineteenth century. Ambiguities surrounding local jurisdiction and prerogative, conflicts over special legislation, competition over political patronage, and prolonged agonizing over the public and private functions of municipal rule greatly troubled state legislators and municipal councils. By the late nineteenth century, state-municipal relations had reached a critical impasse. Local governments issued political and legal challenges to state supremacy over municipal affairs that ultimately crystallized around the home rule movement (Griffith 1974). The approaching municipal revolt had its origins in the antebellum era. The distinguishing characteristics of U.S. local government relative to that of Canada—idiosyncratic municipal legislation and the integration of local governments into patronage politics—interacted in such a way as to hobble both state and local governments and set them against each other (Munro 1923, 1:84–107, 198–233). The dynamics of intergovernmental conflict threw up insurmountable barriers to unifying public and private charity in the localities.

Idiosyncratic municipal legislation became the pattern of municipal rule in colonial times. Before the War of Independence, colonial governors or proprietors exercised royal prerogative in granting municipal charters. These corporations stood beyond legislative interference apart from matters of taxation. Executive prerogative vanished with the Revolution, and state legislatures assumed control over municipal governments. Municipal charters became statutory instruments, and the states could impose charters with or without the consent of the localities. Until the mid–nineteenth century, legislative supremacy was rarely enforced contrary to local interests. Municipal governments normally solicited amendments to their charters, and legislatures obliged. The instruments of rule for cities, towns, villages, and counties evolved piecemeal through idiosyncratic, or special, acts. Over time, this introduced an element of inflexibility into state-local relations that not only subverted municipal autonomy but also failed to compensate for the void in municipal leadership with effective state guidance.

The accretion of special acts made it difficult to mobilize local governments for achieving purposes of general interest to state legislators. Uniform municipal legislation most often conflicted with prior special enactments. This made the judiciary the final arbiters of state-municipal relations. It fell to the courts to decide which law, general or special, superseded the other. New York State's failed attempt to consolidate and rationalize municipal poor relief in 1896 illustrated well this tendency:

> Lack of an integrated policy and of clear definition weakened the effective operation of these statutes. The situation was further complicated by the growth of an unwieldy body of special laws around the two basic poor-relief acts of 1896. At times functions were delegated to new bodies without the repeal of legislation that vested them in existing agencies. Special acts relating exclusively to particular localities and wholesale exemptions in general laws also contributed to the confusion. Some important provisions were hidden away in obscure parts of the statute books. Instances where one statute contradicted another were not rare. Welfare administration on the state level was loosely divided among a growing number of boards, commissions, and similar bodies. On the local level, more than a thousand officers—town overseers of the poor, county superintendents of the poor, magistrates, justices of the peace, city commissioners of charities, and others—were vested with poor-relief responsibilities. (Schneider and Deutsch 1941, 269)

Arbitrating the conflict between general and special law did not provide the only challenge for jurists seeking to reconcile the mass of contradictory legislation regulating municipal governments. Justices were more frequently called upon to rule on inconsistencies between special acts. "No one knows the exact range of powers which appertain at any given moment to any particular city, unless it be the head of the city's legal department," William Bennet Munro remarked in the 1920s, "and even he cannot be sure of his ground. The courts are continually proving by their decisions that even the heads of city legal departments do not know what powers the municipality possesses" (1923, 1:204).

In the mid–nineteenth century, the legislative practice of special enactments combined with patronage politics to make state tutelage of municipal rule even more conflict ridden. When local, state, and national party politics fused, state legislators were frequently willing to amend municipal statutes to advance partisan causes that violated the maxims of local initiative and consent. There were two forces driving state intervention in local affairs—one fiscal and the other constitutional. Normally, both state and local governments primarily drew their income from property taxes. The balance heavily favored the municipalities and presented state and local governments with zero-sum competition over tax revenue. Since municipal offices, contracts, and franchises formed the largest concentrations of political patronage, state legislatures became increasingly tempted to gain control over the strategic assets of municipal rule. States usually crossed local governments in one of two ways. One method was to seize control of a municipal agency and oblige the disenfranchised locality to continue to finance its operation. A second device was to legislate municipal contributions to public improvements under state control. Equally important, constitutional prohibitions against state subsidies to private corporations also induced state legislators to deploy municipal finances in the service of patronage politics. These same constitutional restrictions did not initially bar legislators from mandating local governments to finance privately held corporations. And so, states often circumvented these constitutional provisions with special acts compelling municipal governments to subsidize private companies favored within the legislatures. These practices backfired as local political coalitions banded together to spearhead new constitutional limitations on state authority over municipal finance.

In Canada, provincial-municipal relations markedly departed from state-municipal relations in the United States. Municipal law applied generally from locality to locality, not specifically. Canadian municipalities could not appeal to a tradition of home rule to resist provincial mandates as U.S. local governments could. In any case, the provinces sidestepped local controversies with broad, uniform grants of municipal authority that preempted constant applications for increased powers. Provincial legislators also lacked the range of motivations for special acts that dangled before state legislators. Provincial and municipal politics did not mate. Municipal patronage did not influence the outcome of provincial elections as it did in state elections, and so provincial legislators had no incentives to manage directly the local pork barrel. Nonpartisan municipal councils offered no clear targets for enhancing party fortunes. Further, public finance tended to minimize friction between provincial and local governments as it maximized friction between state and local governments. Tax sharing between provincial and municipal governments was not essential to party patronage. Provincial revenues mainly derived from custom duties before the Confederation of 1867 and from Dominion subsidies thereafter. The provinces financed the most important vehicles of party patronage—the civil service and public works projects—independently of property taxes, which were the mainstay of municipal government.

These contrasting patterns of intergovernmental relationships created differing opportunities for unifying public and private charity in each country. The ease with which the provinces institutionalized municipal subsidies to voluntary hospitals sharply differed from the political controversies surrounding state-mandated financing of private charities. These differences become more comprehensible in light of the discrepant institutional histories of municipal rule. In Canada, uniform municipal statutes afforded the provinces a medium for enlisting local finance for provincial aims. Ontario hospital policy illustrated well this tendency. Mandatory subsidies to voluntary hospitals applied uniformly across all levels of local government. In contemplating the hospital subsidy law, the province risked violating no constitutional law, express or implied, governing provincial-municipal relations. Nor did the legislation risk conflicting with any special acts as no body of idiosyncratic municipal law existed. Compulsory payments to voluntary hospitals occasioned no political backlash. This device had not acquired a disreputable history in Canada whereas U.S. legislators had formerly tainted this class of law with partisan motives, thereby casting a dark shadow over future applications, even meritorious ones.

In the United States, states commonly had no authority to subsidize voluntary hospitals since private charities fell under constitutional prohibitions against special incorporation laws and subsidies to private associations. Further, uniform statutes mandating local subsidies to voluntary hospitals, even if the state legislators were inclined to pass them, would need to surmount a growing range of legal and political obstacles: constitutional law, the judiciary, local governments, and the Protestant charitable establishment. Constitutional amendments eventually stripped state governments of their authority to compel local governments to finance private institutions. The judiciary held the power to interpret which municipal legislation out of the universe of special acts applied in any given circumstances. Municipal resistance to state legislative direction gathered additional force as the United States passed from the Civil War era into the progressive era. And last, the representatives of the Protestant charities concerned with poor relief—the Charity Organization Societies—opposed any merger of public and private charities under government funding and supervision.

The Making and Meaning of Hospital Policy in the Postbellum Era

The first generation of hospital policy emerged in the midst of the progressive era as the foundations of municipal rule underwent their last transformation before the depression. The principles and practices of hospital policy in the United States, as in Canada, represented a confluence of three institutional forces: hospital reform, political reform, and the restoration of the maxims of antebellum poor relief. Reformed hospitals extended their appeal to all social classes. As the self-supporting began to patronize voluntary hospitals with greater frequency, political reformers endeavored to institutionalize nonpartisan and administratively sound methods for underwriting publicly financed hospital charity. The ways and means of U.S. hospital policy drew their inspiration from the historical division of labor between public and private charity that prevailed before the Civil War. Progressive reforms renewed the separation of public charity for the sick poor from the financing and management of private hospitals. The attendant rise of municipally owned and funded hospitals for the poor paralleled the rise of a private, commercial, hospital system for the self-supporting classes. By the onset of the Great Depression, a singular integrative principle of U.S. hospital policy had emerged from the social and political transitions of the late nineteenth and early twentieth centuries: public accommodations for the poor; private arrangements for those of means.

As hospital reform popularized demand for hospital care and fees became the principal source of revenue, hospitals proliferated rapidly. In 1873, the American Medical Association's first hospital census identified 177 hospitals of all kinds. In 1935, the U.S. Business Census reported information on nearly 5,000 acute-care hospitals under AMA registry. Hospitals had completed the break with the past. They were no longer obscure poor relief charities but instead were specialized centers of therapeutic nursing and medical care dotting the landscape of every U.S. city. The transition crowned voluntary hospitals as the dominant institutions of the U.S. hospital industry. Denominational rivalries fueled voluntary hospitals' rise to preeminence. The formation of Catholic charities growing out of midcentury immigration had drawn together Protestant sects to establish and maintain hospital charities. While church-run hospitals normally fell under the management of Catholic nursing orders, Protestant benevolent associations more commonly established nonsectarian hospitals. Confessionally based hospitals controlled almost two-thirds of acute-care beds—more than doubling the accommodations in municipal hospitals and besting provision in for-profit hospitals five times over. U.S. voluntary hospitals derived very little of their income from public subsidies compared to those of Canada. The great majority of voluntary hospital revenue came from paying patients since public funding earmarked for hospital care mostly went to institutions under municipal control. The two-tiered hospital system—one public and reserved for the poor and the other private and primarily devoted to paying patients—owed its origins to the hospital policies of reforming municipal governments.

The transformation of hospital charity coincided with urban political reform. Municipal hospital policies took some of their inspiration from progressive era doctrines of political and administrative betterment. The objects of progressive reform in the United States broadly corresponded to those of Canadian political reform. The aims included leveling the inconsistencies in the legal order that had previously flourished under partisan control over policy making and implementation. Routinizing public financing and regulation implied constructing clearly defined, uniform sets of meanings and purposes to guide policy making. Rationalizing the legal order also called for standardizing the rules and regulations governing public spending and administration. And as had happened in Canada, political reform in the United States sought to achieve these ends by expanding the scope of executive prerogative, consolidating government agencies, centralizing control over public administration, and instituting merit-based civil service reform. However, similar attempts at reform gave rise to opposing policy outcomes in each country. In Canada, the rationalization of hospital policy expanded and formalized public subsidies to voluntary hospitals. In the United States, the rationalization of hospital policy brought widespread government ownership of hospitals in spite of ever-present opportunities to subsidize voluntary hospitals.

The institutional motifs of the antebellum charitable establishment channeled the reform impulse in differing directions in one country and the other. In Canada, renewing publicly sponsored hospital care fused together provincial, municipal, and voluntary endeavors as provincial legislatures remained the undivided sovereigns over hospital charity. In the United States, reaffirming the principles and practices of antebellum poor relief required undivided municipal sovereignty over public charity in the first instance and, second, separating public and private charities into two self-governing, functionally differentiated establishments. First, progressives fought to roll back state regulation of municipal elections, legislation, and budgeting. To lessen partisan influence over local policy making, urban reform was premised on breaking mutually supporting linkages between urban, state, and national party organizations. The immunization of local government from state oversight also came in the form of constitutional and statutory prohibitions against state laws that obliged local governments to raise and spend city taxes on state-sponsored initiatives. Other constitutional amendments made allowances for the granting of home rule—the right of local political coalitions to draft and ratify city charters. Home rule afforded city governments unilateral authority to establish municipal priorities for hospital charity.

The winning of municipal sovereignty over public charity was the essential first step toward restoring the antebellum charitable establishment. The second challenge was to separate public from private charity. For progressive reformers, public subsidies to private charities were aberrations to be avoided or abolished. Giving to some private charities was thought to encourage all of them to resort to the public trough. Therefore, petitions for municipal assistance would become endemic features of policy making and complicate the task of ridding municipal government of influence peddling and patronage politics. Public financing for hospital charity confined to municipally owned institutions promised "economy" and "efficiency" since only public agencies could be completely brought under the discipline of the municipal executive. Urban political reformers found common cause with the politically mobilized representatives of the Protestant charitable establishment—the Charity Organization Societies (COS). Since the COS upbraided public charity for inducing poverty in the first instance, they vehemently attacked public subsidies to private charities. As the argument went, public subsidies caused an oversupply of private charities and defeated COS efforts to scale back charity giving. In addition to blaming public subsidies for creating needless duplication of charities, the COS held them responsible for advancing the fortunes of "politically influential and irresponsible charity givers"—bywords for Catholic charities—over those of the "scientific charities"—the moniker for Protestant-run charities.

Urban reformers sponsored major investments in public hospitals and sought to eradicate public financing of private hospitals in the name of restoring the modus vivendi of the antebellum charitable establishment. The renewed separation of public and private charity engendered a new synthesis of meanings and practices specific to hospital policy. Municipal hospitals would confine their services to the poor rather than operate for community-wide benefit. If public hospitals attempted to attract paying patients, it would violate the boundary between public and private hospitals. The newfound, sacred domain of voluntary hospitals was the pay-patient trade. The socioeconomic transformation of voluntary hospitals combined with the inauguration of municipal hospitals for the poor to institutionalize a two-tiered, class-stratified hospital industry. In the progressive era, public arrangements for the poor and private provisions for the working population emerged as the paradigm of U.S. hospital policy.

The Derogation of State Government: New York

Developments in New York State again serve as a useful comparison to those in the Canadian provinces. New York was atypical of U.S. states. It came closest to institutionalizing the key components of provincial hospital policies in Canada: state funding of private charities, state-mandated contributions from local governments to voluntary hospitals, and uniform supervision of all local charities, public and private. Events in the Empire State illustrated well the unraveling of state authority over local charity, the restoration of municipal sovereignty over publicly sponsored hospital care, and the impact of progressive doctrines on hospital policies.

The New York electorate had approved a sweeping constitutional amendment prohibiting state funding of private corporations as early as 1846 that, in principle, should have precluded state subsidies to private charities issued upon the authority of the Commissioners of Emigration before the Civil War. While these payments went overlooked in the antebellum period, state subsidies were discontinued in the early 1870s. In a series of court rulings, the New York judiciary pieced together a poor-law doctrine that effectively barred the state from extending any direct assistance to local charities beyond payments to poor-law officials for the care of state paupers. In their deliberations the courts reasoned that general poor relief fell within the exclusive jurisdiction of the municipalities under New York constitutional and statutory law, a historically accurate, if not farsighted, view. The courts exempted certain charities from the no-state-subsidy rule, namely, institutions for the blind, the deaf, and juvenile delinquents, on the conviction that these organizations relieved a statewide, as opposed to a specifically local, clientele. And, state assistance had proven to be a practical necessity. A 1874 constitutional amendment subsequently converted the court's view on the matter into fundamental law (Lincoln 1906, 680–83).

The injunction against direct state subsidies to private charities left open the question of whether the state could regulate by other means the public financing of local charities, in particular, whether the state possessed the authority to legislate municipal contributions to private charities. New York's constitution forbade both state and local governments from voting public moneys to private enterprises. But like the vast majority of state constitutions, New York law permitted municipalities to subsidize private charities in making provision for the poor. Further, the constitution did not address the possibility of state-legislated contributions from municipal governments to private charities in exacting terms. Municipalities, of their own accord and under state mandates, subsidized both private orphanages on a large scale in the last half of the nineteenth century and, to a lesser extent than child-saving institutions, general and specialty hospitals. Compared to the local subsidies to hospitals in other states however, New York's voluntary hospitals received extensive subsidies from municipalities, especially in New York City (Barbour et al. 1901, 123).

Several controversies over state-mandated contributions to private charities in Brooklyn provided the backdrop for restraining the state's hand in governing local subsidies. One such scandal concerned a state law that earmarked local taxes for distribution to private charities in Brooklyn. The city had subsidized its voluntary hospitals since the 1840s. Voluntary hospitals came to disagree with the city about the size of the subsidy in the 1880s and appealed to the state legislature to enforce their claims against the municipal purse. Brooklyn's hospital boards successfully lobbied the state legislature to bring the annual subsidy from the municipal treasury to $4,000 per hospital. In total, fifteen of Brooklyn's seventeen hospitals benefited from the state law, which covered a third of their collective operating expenses.

The state law embarrassed a city administration widely lauded for its progressive reforms and generated contempt for state oversight of municipal government. The sponsors of the law attempted no elementary distinctions between the hospitals included in the subsidy list. Small hospitals dispensing little charity received the same amount as large ones. In 1890, the governor heeded the pleas of Brooklyn's reform mayor, Seth Low, and vetoed changes to the law that would have brought more hospitals into the system (Pilcher 1890). The event snowballed into an 1894 constitutional amendment forbidding the state to legislate local subsidies to private charities, neatly dovetailing with earlier court rulings that outlawed state efforts to compel municipal corporations to take stock in private enterprises (Lincoln 1906, 683–86). For Brooklyn however, the constitution provided no immediate protection from the existing state mandate. The older subsidy law was grandfathered, making new subsidies illegal but leaving the old ones to be amended at the state's discretion. Thus, state-mandated subsidies to private charities in Brooklyn continued until 1898 when Brooklyn was absorbed into the larger metropolitan government of New York City.

Now that the state no longer possessed the power to marshal state or municipal financing of local charity, all that remained in its arsenal for regulating private charity was the State Board of Charities. Founded in 1867, the board originally confined its investigations to state-owned and state-assisted charities, prisons excepted. State laws of 1873, and later an 1894 constitutional amendment, empowered the board to supervise any charity in the state, public or private, the widest grant of authority bestowed upon any such agency in the United States. Further, any charities seeking incorporation would have to obtain approval from the board, making New York the only state to regulate the incorporation of private charities before the depression. Ultimately, the board entered the twentieth century with fewer supervisory powers than anticipated. After the board suffered prolonged resistance to state supervision from private charities, legal and political challenges to the its authority in the 1890s whittled down its mandate. In *People ex rel. State Charities Board v. New York Society for Prevention of Cruelty to Children,* the society called upon the New York Supreme Court to furnish a definition of charity that would exempt the society from state supervision. The judgment offered a definition of charity that limited the power of the board to inspect government-owned or publicly subsidized charities only, releasing unassisted private charities from any state regulation:

> This corporation has been given legal capacity to take and administer gifts and bequests that would be called charitable under the Statute of Elizabeth, and under the general rules of law applicable to trusts, colleges, academies, and nearly all institutions of a learning or of a literary character, and even cities, villages and other municipal corporations, may take and administer such gifts, but that fact cannot in the least affect their true character, or convert them into charitable institutions. The scheme of state supervision was not intended to apply to every institution engaged in some good or commendable work for the relief of humanity from some of the various ills with which it is afflicted, but only to those maintained in whole or in part by the state or some of its political divisions, through which charity, as such, was dispensed by public authority to those having a claim upon the generosity or bounty of the state. It will exclude only those institutions that ask nothing in the form of charity from the state. This system of state supervision does not extend to the efforts of private benevolence since the government is no way connected with it. (*People ex rel. State Charities Board v. New York Society for Prevention of Cruelty to Children,* 55 N.E. 1063, 161 N.Y. 233 [1900])

As illustrated here, sovereignty over hospital policy greatly differed between U.S. states and Canadian provinces at the turn of the century. New York State had no legal authority to subsidize voluntary hospitals and could only offer payments to local governments for the hospital care of those defined as the state poor, not local patients. Canadian provinces extended subsidies to all voluntary and municipal hospitals on behalf of any patient who could not pay the full hospital rate. New York State had no constitutional warrant to mandate local subsidies to private charities. Canadian provinces drafted uniform municipal legislation compelling all local governments to contribute to the expenses of provincially recognized hospitals operating within their jurisdictions. State supervision extended to public charities and to private charities in receipt of municipal subsidies, and so local governments primarily defined the nature and extent of state hospital regulation. Canadian provinces solely determined which hospitals came under public supervision. In Canada, the provinces were the sovereigns of hospital policy. In the United States, the municipalities were paramount.

The Restoration of Municipal Sovereignty: New York City
Charity, Regulated

To understand how municipal governments came to formulate the first generation of hospital policy in the United States, the following analysis once again considers the case most similar to that of Canada to demonstrate the political dynamics separating the two countries. New York City experienced and experimented with the core elements of Canadian hospital policy. The city came under state mandates to subsidize private charities. Local officials independently established per-diem reimbursements to voluntary hospitals for public dependents. And, the city's Department of Charities devised a system of public supervision for all hospitals that came into receipt of municipal payments. Nonetheless, New York City retreated from subsidizing private hospitals to construct the United States' largest public hospital system. For municipal reformers, the establishment and maintenance of hospitals under direct ownership and control of the city were integral components of a broader campaign to dampen partisan influence over municipal politics. Progressives viewed the giving of public subsidies to private charities as a lineal descendant of the spoils system or, at the very least, as a constant temptation for politicians to implicate subsidy privileges in electioneering. Public money for public institutions only was the popular cry of municipal reformers who sought to prevent private charities from encircling and dominating the development of municipal charity giving. The following summary of the New York City hospital reforms condenses the detailed accounts entailed in Bird Coler's *Municipal Subsidies to Private Charities* (1899) and *Municipal Government* (1901). At the turn of the century, Coler was the New York City comptroller, a voting member of the powerful Board of Estimate and Apportionment, and the architect of New York City's reformed public charities.

When the charter of greater New York came into effect in 1898, municipal subsidies to private charities absorbed three-fifths of New York City's $5 million relief budget, a marked departure from the early apportionment of city spending on public and private charity. At midcentury, when the public charitable establishment greatly overshadowed New York City's private relief societies, the city paid less than $10,000 to private charities out of its $430,000 charity budget. Within the space of thirty years however, private relief organizations came to administer over one-half of the city's $2.7 million annual relief appropriation, and in 1898, city payments to private charities surpassed total charity spending for 1880, over $3 million. New York City's private charities had risen above their humble origins as adjuncts to the city's charities to become the major shareholder of municipal relief funds in a little less than fifty years.

As in Brooklyn, municipal subsidies to private charities exploded in the 1870s, 1880s, and 1890s in New York City. Both cities deeply cut their relief expenditures, among other costs, to balance the municipal budget so as to restore the confidence of their principal creditors. Outdoor relief terminated in the 1870s, save for the distribution of coal to the poor in New York City. Capital improvements were withheld from the assorted public charities: two dozen almshouses, orphanages, pesthouses, and hospitals. Municipal retrenchment did not reduce the need for charitable assistance. Rather, the need shifted onto private charities. The irony was that the cities inadvertently funded the aggrandizement of private charities, nullifying the projected savings of municipal restraint. Private charities appealed to the state for assistance after their pleas for aid met with indifference locally. Even though the state could not legally advance any of its own capital, legislators pledged city money to those claiming to be surrogates for municipal charity. The city voted on less than $100,000 of the $3.1 million turned over to private charities from the city relief budget in 1898. The balance was distributed at the behest of the state.

The state subsidy law for New York City fell prey to the same criticisms leveled against that of Brooklyn. State legislators had not calibrated the lump-sum grants to the volume and nature of services provided for the ostensible benefit of the city by private charities. Municipal authorities had not entered into the political bargaining that prefaced subsidy legislation, and further, the subsidy law did not vest the city with any residual authority over the administration of the funds. The municipality did not gain any right to inspect, audit, or otherwise regulate charities receiving city aid. The state's mandatory subsidy acts, in theory, could have remained a permanent component of the New York City budget into the twentieth century. The 1894 constitutional amendment forbidding such legislation applied to subsequent, not prior, enactments, and the New York City laws, like that of Brooklyn, predated 1894.

The reform administration that carried the 1898 municipal election launched a campaign to release the city from existing state mandates and to overhaul public relief according to the latest theories of political and administrative betterment. Bird Coler spearheaded the movement to restore municipal autonomy in the affairs of public charity. Before approaching the state to have the New York and Brooklyn subsidy laws repealed, Coler sought out and obtained the backing of national, state, and local charity organizations: the National Conference on Charities and Corrections, the New York State Board of Charities, the New York State Charities Aid Association, and the Charity Organization Society of the City of New York. With the weight of informed and respected opinion behind him, Coler prevailed upon the chairman of the Senate Committee on Cities, Senator Stranahan, to have the subsidy laws voided. The Stranahan Bill, passed in 1899, recognized the undivided authority of the city's Board of Estimate and Apportionment in determining relief appropriations to private charities and closed the door to any subsequent state mandates.

Coler had played upon the indignant sentiments of New York's Protestant charitable establishment to win exclusive control over the city's charity budget but considered it an impossible task to satisfy calls for the complete abolition of public subsidies to private charities. Coler's advocates equated prolonging subsidies with institutionalizing political bargaining between the city and private charities that bordered on corruption. Subsidies would ostensibly undermine any attempt to unify and rationalize public administration. Public finance should be wholly controlled by public officials and, therefore, spent on institutions owned and operated by the city. Coler claimed that these conclusions were theoretically sound but practically unfeasible. The city's own institutions had suffered neglect, leaving them insufficient to master the needs for public relief. Coler was alive to the importance of maintaining the strength of publicly assisted private charities. Many provided critical services for the city and would likely suffer needless hardship or cease operations if the city brought funding to an abrupt end. Coler cautioned the abolitionists to prepare for less than total victory. For the good of the city and private charity, subsidies would survive the approaching shake-up of municipal finance.

Coler devised a strategy to reconcile the demands for reform with the inescapable reality of private charities' dependence on municipal financing. In 1900, the city introduced a regulatory framework that went as far as possible in the direction of progressive reform without living up to the progressive ideal of eliminating subsidies entirely. Coler implemented two key reforms that met the essential tests of public accountability. First, the city put all subsidy appropriations on budget. Some subsidy payments under the old dispensation had been financed through special excise funds that lay outside the orbit of public scrutiny. Coler discontinued the practice. Second, the city instituted common features of the subsidy laws governing the distribution of public funding in Canada: per-diem disbursements, graduated according to the nature of services provided and applied uniformly to all institutions of the same class, and an allowance for public inspection and audit. Private charities would henceforth demonstrate competent service to inmates and probity in their bookkeeping to qualify for public subsidies. Further, the Board of Estimate expanded the city's corps of inspectors to monitor the circumstances of all patients for whom private charities would seek reimbursements.

The reconstitution of the city's subsidy program began to strip public appropriations of their earlier identification with political corruption, and so the friction surrounding them lessened considerably. Further, the new subsidy policy had an unintended benefit. It afforded city officials an extremely flexible instrument for long-term planning and managing short-term crisis. The city only needed to decide upon a prospective balance between the share of the budget earmarked for public charities and that dispensed to private relief agencies and then fine-tune the regulations governing subsidies to gradually conform public spending to projected targets. Likewise, during times of crisis, subsidies to private charities could be quickly and responsibly liberalized to alleviate excessive pressures upon the city's own institutions.

Coler had advertised subsidy regulation as making the best of a bad situation, as an interim policy to be discarded with the establishment of public institutions capable of handling the city's poor-law obligations without private assistance. The irony confronting the city was that the very subsidy policy it introduced for the purposes of defending and restoring the budgets of public charities gave municipal officials a responsible system for extending further assistance to private charities. The city took time to decide which of these tendencies to follow. In 1899, the year before the new subsidy policy went into effect, the city was working against the inertia of high spending on private charities. The option to continue the practice was not without advocates. New York City hospital luminary S. S. Goldwater, the superintendent of Mount Sinai Hospital, argued as much when he characterized as unwarranted further investments in municipal hospitals insofar as the city's voluntary hospitals could put over ten thousand beds at the disposal of the Department of Charities.

> The humanitarian object of gratuitous hospital support is the proper care of poor and helpless sick persons; from the standpoint of the taxpayer it is the proper care of such persons *at the minimum public costs.* If, therefore, privately managed hospitals are able to care for their partially subsidized patients quite as well as such patients are cared for in hospitals supported wholly by public funds (a supposition which I think will be accepted without question) it would seem to be sound civic and business policy for the tax-payer to unite with the private hospital to further the development of the system. The pur-

pose of appropriations is everywhere the same, namely, to encourage
private philanthropic endeavor and thus to lighten the burdens of the
local government . . . of its responsibility for the care of the indigent
sick. (Goldwater 1909, 244–45)

Contrary to Goldwater's hopes, municipal spending on voluntary hospitals declined precipitously between the 1900 subsidy reform and the onset
of the depression in order to free up city money for the construction of
municipal hospitals. When Coler first proposed to revolutionize the relationship between the city and private charities in 1899, New York City's
nine hospitals attended to a largely undifferentiated clientele of chronic,
contagious, and acute cases. These hospitals often performed several other
custodial functions as well as serving as a haven for the sick poor. For
example, Children's Hospital on Blackwell's Island reported an average
stay per inmate approaching eight months, more akin to the profile of an
orphanage than that of a hospital like the City's Infant Hospital, where the
average stay fell just short of three months, or City Hospital, one month.
Thirty years later, the city possessed the nation's largest municipal hospital
system, encompassing twenty-three hospitals with clearly defined missions—twelve general hospitals, two allied specialty hospitals, eight contagious diseases hospitals, and one mental hospital—and service patterns
much more closely approximating those of the private hospitals. Depriva-
tizing the city's hospital budget made possible the large-scale growth and
transformation of municipal hospital service (table 3.1). Payments to private hospitals dropped from nearly one-half to less than one-seventh of the
municipal hospital care budget between 1899 and 1930, only to be reinvig-
orated slightly by the economic crises of the depression. The proportion of
public charge days given in public and voluntary hospitals followed a similar pattern (table 3.2). The new subsidy regime reversed the shrinking of the
public hospital system relative to that of voluntary hospitals, and the
expansion of municipal hospitals matched private hospital growth during
the first three decades of the twentieth century (table 3.3).

Municipal governments in other important mid-Atlantic cities like
Washington, DC, and Baltimore had placed themselves in a comparable
situation to that of New York City, and they also tapered public subsidies
to private hospitals in order to establish and expand public hospitals
exclusively dedicated to caring for the poor (Kingsdale 1981, 82–248;
Warner et al. 1935, 186–87). In Pennsylvania, the state had become the primary source of government subsidies to voluntary hospitals in addition to
owning and managing many hospitals. Political reforms there in the 1920s
also borrowed from the example of New York City (Frankel 1925; Stevens
1984). For voluntary hospitals, costs mounted while public subsidies were

TABLE 3.1.   New York City Expenditures on Hospital Charity, 1899, 1910, 1930, 1934

	Total (in thousands)	In Public Hospitals	In Voluntary Hospitals	Subsidies as a Percentage of Voluntary Hospital Income
1899	1,575	822 (52)	753 (48)	17.5
1910	4,051	2,761 (69)	1,290 (31)	16.0
1930	17,607	14,952 (85)	2,655 (15)	6.4
1934	23,893	19,300 (81)	4,593 (19)	13.2

Source: Coler 1899, 23–32; Jones and Thomas 1938, 3:419–71; New York State Board of Charities 1900, 2:1396–1408; U.S. Bureau of the Census 1913, 322–30.
Note: Percentages are given in parentheses.

TABLE 3.2.   Patient Days and Public Charge Days in New York City Hospitals, 1899, 1906, 1934

	Total (in thousands)	In Public Hospitals	In Voluntary Hospitals
Patient Days			
1899	2,571	1,229 (48)	1,342 (52)
1934	11,865	5,692 (48)	6,173 (52)
Public Charge Days			
1906	2,240	1,252 (56)	988 (44)
1934	7,488	5,692 (76)	1,796 (24)

Source: See Table 3.3.
Note: Percentages are given in parentheses.

TABLE 3.3.   Beds in New York City Hospitals, 1899, 1910, 1934

	Public Hospitals	Voluntary Hospitals	Total Beds	In Public Hospitals	In Voluntary Hospitals
1899	9	86	—	—	—
1910	13	90	20,437	8,394 (41)	12,043 (59)
1934	23	104	36,056	14,849 (41)	21,207 (59)

Source: Goldwater 1909, 11:271–72; Jones and Thomas 1938, 3:419–71; New York State Board of Charities 1900, 2:1396–1408; U.S. Bureau of the Census 1913, 322–30.
Note: Percentages are given in parentheses.

entirely lacking or diminishing in the early, critical years of the twentieth century. Private hospitals reduced their commitments to charity and redirected the poor to the growing public hospital establishment. In some urban areas, subsidies to private hospitals lingered as supplements to public hospital care as had happened in New York City. Nonetheless, voluntary hospitals primarily reoriented their services to the needs of paying patients. The opportunity had passed for achieving universal access to hospital care with comprehensive subsidy policies.

The United States' Two-Tiered Hospital System

The United States developed two distinct hospital systems in the postbellum era, one public, and the other private (table 3.4). These hospital systems were differentiated by ownership, financing, clientele, and public accountability. Public hospitals primarily descended from the municipal poorhouses. They were overwhelmingly devoted to the care of poor, derived their financing from municipal taxes, and were nominally subject to state supervision. By 1936, public hospitals accounted for about one-quarter of acute-care beds. Municipal hospitals tended to cluster in urban centers and were usually impressive edifices; the average number of beds in public hospitals nearly doubled that of voluntary hospitals. Voluntary, nonprofit hospitals dominated the private hospital system. They rose to preeminence on fees from self-supporting patients. In aggregate, U.S. voluntary hospitals gathered approximately 10 percent of income from public sources, far less than Canadian voluntary hospitals derived from the provincial subsidy laws. In the 1920s, the fragments of the subsidy laws surviving the political adversity of the progressive era encompassed less than one-third of all voluntary hospitals (U.S. Bureau of the Census 1925, 26). New York City's voluntary hospitals comprised a large fraction of the eight hundred hospitals aided and supervised by local and state authorities across the United States. But, the large majority of private hospitals had never come under any formal public supervision, and very few had experienced any substantive government regulation.

Public hospitals did not appear everywhere. They concentrated in urban areas as did most hospital construction (table 3.5). Outside of the cities, many county overseers continued the practice of setting aside space in local almshouses as sickness wards. Many others constructed freestanding poor-law infirmaries that did not become designated as hospitals in official records. Another common practice in counties without public hospitals was to make contractual arrangements with municipal hospitals in adjoining counties, with state hospitals for the poor, or with state-owned hospitals affiliated with public medical schools. Yet another practice was to purchase care from local private hospitals—nonprofit and profit making—where economies of scale also did not warrant constructing free-standing public hospitals (Agnew 1935, 892). In the first decades of the twentieth century, the great majority of public spending for hospital care, over 70 percent, went to municipal hospitals in the most densely populated areas in the United States. Urban counties and city governments routinely built public hospitals in the midst of abundant opportunities to support

TABLE 3.4.   Hospital Capacity and Financing, by Ownership,
United States, 1935

	Public	Voluntary	Profit	Total
Number of hospitals	569	2,469	1,542	4,580
Number of beds	103,269 (26)	249,758 (63)	45,632 (11)	398,659
Average number of beds				
per hospital	181	101	30	87
Admissions				
(in thousands)	1,449 (24)	3,822 (64)	719 (12)	5,990
Patient days				
(in thousands)	26,119 (35)	43,115 (57)	6,262 (8)	75,496
Mean stay in days	18	11	9	12.6
Occupancy	79	55	41	60
Source of Income	%	%	%	%
Taxes	81.1	10.2	4.1	23.8
Pay patients	16.7	70.8	91.4	62.4
Endowments and gifts	2.2	19.0	4.5	13.8

Source: Mountin, Pennell, and Flook 1938, 12; Pennell, Mountin, and Hankla 1938, 15.
Note: Nonfederal, short-term general, and allied specialty hospitals of AMA registry that omitted 1,491 unregistered hospitals, representing about 6% of the nation's capacity. Percentages are given in parentheses.

TABLE 3.5.   Incidence of Public and Private Hospitals, by County and
Population, United States, 1936

	Public Only	Private Only	Both	None	Total
Counties	154 (5)	1,321 (43)	296 (10)	1,302 (42)	3,073
Percentage of					
U.S. population	3	36	46	15	100

Source: Data from American Hospital Association and American Public Welfare Association 1938, 8:155.
Note: Nonfederal, short-term general, and allied specialty hospitals. Percentages are given in parentheses.

the sick poor in voluntary hospitals. Municipal hospitals clustered in urban counties—less than 10 percent of all counties—but encompassing about one-half of the population.

The rise of the municipal hospital system was not a foregone conclusion of the rationalization of publicly sponsored hospital charity. Even though the poor laws called upon local governments to provide for the sick poor, establishing public hospitals represented only one of several alternatives for fulfilling this obligation. No mandate to build hospitals inhered in U.S. poor laws (U.S. Bureau of the Census 1914). Constitutions generally prevented state governments from subsidizing private charities but did not prohibit municipalities from doing so in all but a very few states. Apart from the permissive legal context, subsidies to voluntary hospitals had advantages. The economic incentives were often favorable. Establishing public hospitals—even in those cases where local governments renovated the existing physical plant of almshouses—generally entailed substantial capital costs. Contracting out public charges to voluntary hospitals often promised a reduction in both overhead and direct operating costs. Taxpayers might be convinced that the wasteful political jobbery connected with so many public institutions could be altogether eliminated through public subsidies and, perhaps, gratified to know that private institutions could better attend to the moral and spiritual needs of charity recipients. Further, municipal hospitals did not perform any essential role in deterring charity abuse that could not have been combined with subsidies to private hospitals. As happened in New York City, recipients of public charity cared for in voluntary hospitals did not evade the disgrace of city almoners inquiring into their financial and personal affairs. Moreover, there was nothing intrinsic to municipal ownership that abetted the professed aims of reform under the progressive banner: the strengthening of the executive prerogative; improved public accountability for local government spending; the lessening of partisan influence over local policy making; and finally, standardizing municipal regulations governing publicly sponsored hospital care for the poor. Each of these laudable political reforms could have been easily satisfied in carefully devised subsidy policies as they were in Canada, New York City, and many other U.S. cities.

So why did U.S. city governments commit so many more resources to building, equipping, and operating hospitals than to subsidizing private hospitals when both methods could have satisfied the stated goals of reform? Municipal hospitals symbolized the restoration of the defining practices and principles of antebellum poor relief: municipal sovereignty over public charity and also the separation of the public and private charitable establishments. Local subsidies to private charities were doubly condemned as the case of New York aptly demonstrated. First, subsidies were identified with unprecedented state incursions upon municipal autonomy. Second, they violated the Protestant ethos that suffused both public charity and private philanthropy even as it celebrated the division of labor between the two. The principal allies of progressive reformers were not the arriviste Catholic charities. The political arms of the Protestant charitable establishment—the Charity Organization Societies—were the main proponents of separating public and private charity. Protestants did not much waver in their determination to fashion public services—educational and charitable—into instruments of cultural assimilation. Protestant nativism fueled the tendency to channel public finance into publicly controlled institutions and away from private institutions—even forgoing public spending on charities under Protestant control—to prevent subsidies from assisting minority ethnic groups to secure an institutional basis for cultural self-preservation. In the United States, public subsidies to private charities were constructed as a form of political corruption. Not so in Canada. There, denominational pluralism did not emerge from the arrival of fragmented immigrant minorities but from the union of two evenly matched ethnic blocs with their own established churches. Government patronage of confessionally based charities became politically normalized and rationalized. And, provincial sovereignty over municipal corporations was explicit. Provincially mandated contributions from local governments to private charities did not violate any canons of the Canadian political order. In the United States, public hospitals were tangible monuments to the political success of urban reformers who sought to return municipal governments to their former selves.

Conclusion

The paradigm of U.S. hospital policy drew inspiration from the antebellum charitable establishment. The incipient sovereignty of local governments over poor relief and the exclusive identification of public charity with the bodily sufferings of the poor crowned municipal almshouses as the loci of institutional care for the sick. In the colonial era and the earliest years of the new republic, the predominance of nonconformist Protestant sects in the religious life of the nation made evangelical and educational pursuits the primary objects of private philanthropy. This division of labor among public and private charity gathered additional force with constitutional reforms that divested state governments of their residual sovereignty over private charities and that subsequently dismantled state oversight of municipal poor relief. The reigning orthodoxy of the antebellum charitable establishment was that secular and confessional charities constituted functionally differentiated, noncompetitive, and self-governing complements to one another. In spirit and in law, the finances and management of the two branches were to remain separate. In the United States, public and private charity would not operate in unison.

The postbellum era witnessed profound changes in the scale and scope of private charity and in the meanings and practices associated with publicly sponsored hospital care. The settling of Catholic populations arising out of midcentury immigration produced the denominational rivalries necessary to initiate widespread Protestant involvement in poor relief—a stunning departure from antebellum patterns of confessional philanthropy. The resulting proliferation of private charities intersected with the social and economic transformation of hospital enterprises to make voluntary hospitals the dominant institutions within the industry. Private provisions for the acute sick overtook public accommodations. Correspondingly, local governments were now confronted with two alternatives for fulfilling their obligations to the sick poor: construct and finance public hospitals or subsidize private hospital charities. The latter approach, as local governments discovered, generated intense controversy and sustained political counteroffensives. The settling of the hospital question took its political thrust from an alliance of progressive urban reformers and the representatives of the Protestant charitable establishment. Each party was bent on restoring the principles of the antebellum charitable establishment—the separation and differentiation of public and private charity—within a new matrix of institutional practices. Urban governments reconstituted publicly sponsored care for the sick poor in freestanding, special-purpose hospitals for the poor, notwithstanding the scattered vestiges of public subsidies to private hospitals. Voluntary hospitals were given rights to the pay-patient trade. The resulting two-tiered hospital system became the institutional basis of the emergent paradigm of U.S. hospital policy: public, tax-supported arrangements for the sick poor set apart from the private institutions and economies of hospital care for the self-supporting.

CHAPTER 4

Reconstructing the Public Hospital Economy

The political economy of the Canadian hospital establishment veered toward another transformation with the coming of the depression. The elaboration of a new standard for publicly financed hospital benefits, as with the emergence of the first generation of hospital policy, represented a convergence of three institutional forces: hospital reform, political reform, and historical precedent. The reigning assumption of the pre-depression hospital order was that government-mandated subsidies on behalf of those who could not afford any or all of the costs of their treatment, when added to contributions from paying patients and other private subscriptions, would endow public hospitals with sufficient reserves to provide for all in need of their care. The declining importance of donated labor and capital, the mounting expense of refinements to hospital building codes, and steep advances in hospital-based technologies all pointed to converting hospital finance to the medium of insurance. The urgency of expanding the revenue base of the public hospitals, and its corollary, a dying faith in the virtues of individual responsibility for hospital fees, begat a painstaking reexamination of hospital policy.

At issue was the deceptively simple question of whether collectivizing the financial burdens of individuals' unforeseen hospital stays was more appropriately a matter of public or private initiative. In the 1930s and early 1940s, the general presumption was that social insurance would inevitably carry the heavy freight of the reformed hospital economy. The initial premise of legislative deliberations was that mandatory contributions to health plans under the direction of the provincial governments would serve as the fundaments of prepaid health benefits, and publicly financed hospital schemes did prevail in four provinces before the arrival of national hospital reform. However, there was a private alternative to broad-based, tax-supported hospital insurance that became more salient in the late 1940s and early 1950s—after the federal and provincial governments had conspicuously failed to come to an agreement on a national health plan at the 1945 Dominion-Provincial Conference on Postwar Reconstruction. Industrial relations in Canada approximated those of the United States (Jamieson 1957). Canadian labor laws, tax codes, and union organization all favored the emergence of corporate-financed hospital insurance as an employment fringe benefit. In six provinces, passing consideration was also given to solemnizing a mixed hospital economy: privately funded, employment-based coverage for workers and their dependents and government-sponsored programs for those excluded from the commerce of the voluntary health plans.

The imperative of hospital reform, and its associated controversies, coincided with political reforms that further complicated efforts to modernize hospital policy. Under the old dispensation, the legalities of publicly financed hospital care were uniquely provincial constructs. The gradual erosion of the political and constitutional barriers to federal initiatives in jurisdictions assigned to the provinces multiplied the political channels for generating legislative priorities in the field of hospital regulation. The Canadian parliament became a separate locus for debate over health reform in addition to the provincial legislatures. And a third, extraparliamentary forum for reconciling provincial and national policy making—regularly scheduled federal-provincial conferences of first ministers—was the principal vehicle for reaching intergovernmental accords on major advances for social insurance. The provinces held a veto over federal intervention into health care finance, and provincial opposition to the initial terms and conditions of federal proposals for a national health plan temporarily frustrated progress on hospital reform. The privilege of dismissing federal overtures also imposed an obligation on the provincial governments to steer federal efforts, and their collective determination to exact federal subsidies for hospital care would eventually yield a national mandate for universal hospital insurance. In stark contrast, federal legislators in the United States devised national standards for publicly financed hospital benefits without any direction from state governments.

The weight of institutional precedent ultimately settled the uncertainties and controversies attending national hospital reform. The long-standing maxim of provincial hospital law—universal access to the public hospital system—translated into an abiding concern for universalizing hospital insurance, and the two became synonymous. The 1955 federal-provincial conference became the specific venue for opening negotiations over federal cost sharing of provincially administered hospital insurance. Before that, federal promotions of other social legislation had obscured hospital policy as a distinct focus of national attention. Moreover, the earliest attempts at health reform had envisaged government-sponsored plans for hospital and medical care as jointly insured services. The greater challenge of appeasing the medical profession had overshadowed consideration of separate advances for publicly financed hospital benefits. In the late 1940s and early 1950s, as Canadian doctors withdrew their support for compulsory medical insurance, provincial reformers began to concentrate on mending the public hospital economy. The intransigence of the medical lobbies reinstated the division between hospital and medical policy in the provincial legislatures. Correspondingly, national deliberations over federal grants-in-aid of the provinces for health insurance also severed hospital from medical care. The margin of victory for a nationwide system of universal hospital insurance came from an alliance of provincial governments set on routinizing federal investments in the public hospital system. The governing consensus among them was that hospital care should be allocated on the basis of medical need.

The Long Contretemps

The hospital subsidy laws survived the depression and World War II without far-reaching amendment. Mounting spending on relief, and then the extraordinary demands upon the public fisc stemming from the mobilization, largely distracted Canadian governments from the cause of hospital reform. With the conclusion of the war and the return to prosperity, Canadian legislators would uniquely confront the task of reconstructing the public hospital economy. The immediate response to the crisis in hospital finance was to liberalize the subsidy rates to meet increasing demand for free and low-cost care. Further, provincial and local governments commonly resorted to special allowances to cancel the debts of public hospitals. In the two most populous provinces—Ontario and Quebec—combined provincial-municipal subsidies climbed from under 25 percent of public hospital income in 1928 to 36 percent and 40 percent respectively in 1936 (table 4.1). In the majority of provinces no conscious decision to reform the subsidy laws accompanied rising public spending on hospital charity. However, there were grave doubts as to whether existing arrangements still offered a realistic solution to the problem of hospital finance.

Many of the complaints surrounding the subsidy laws had their origins in the 1920s, even though the depression added a sense of urgency to them. One problem derived from flat-rate, per-diem reimbursements. The provinces introduced the per-diem rates when the sophistication of public hospitals was relatively uniform. As the technological gap widened between the more advanced, urban hospitals and the smaller, rural hospitals, the flat per-diem rates threatened to undermine the rough parity between public service and public compensation. Municipal financing of hospital care also attracted controversy. The causes had less to do with municipal thrift than with escalating hospital fees. In Ontario for example, local-government subsidies exceeded provincial allowances after World War I. Whereas the province accepted reimbursement claims on the basis of hospital billing records, municipal governments more commonly investigated the finances of patients for whom the hospitals were seeking compensation. Public hospitals often referred all nonpaying and part-paying accounts to the local authorities. The municipalities normally accepted responsibility for the poor and the working poor. Judicial constructions of Ontario hospital law made local governments liable for the hospital bills of patients for whom such charges would likely constitute an unreasonable hardship (Cox 1951, 34). But the hardships of poverty-stricken and middle-income patients became more difficult to distinguish as hospital costs overtook the means of wage earners who were otherwise self-supporting. Even though local governments did not break with precedent in refusing to compensate for every unpaid hospital charge, the volume of delinquent accounts soared in the 1930s. This aggravated tensions between distressed local governments and public hospitals, despite rising contributions from municipal budgets for hospital charity (Canadian Hospital Council 1937, 49–64). Laboring under difficulties, some cumulative and others specific to the depression, the subsidy laws remained flexible enough to keep the public hospitals solvent throughout the decade.

TABLE 4.1.   Government Subsidies to Public Hospitals in Select Canadian Provinces, 1936

	Provincial Subsidies (in thousands)	Municipal Subsidies (in thousands)	Combined Government Subsidies (in thousands)	Total Hospital Income (in thousands)
British Columbia	934	628	1,562	3,854
Ontario	1,353	3,042	4,395	12,012
Quebec	3,177	875	4,052	10,124
Saskatchewan	762	68	830	3,485
As a Percentage of Public Hospital Income[a]				
British Columbia	24	16	41	
Ontario	11	25	37	
Quebec	31	9	40	
Saskatchewan	22	2	24	

Source: Ontario 1938, table 18; British Columbia 1938, 90–91; Saskatchewan 1938, 70–71; Quebec 1914–40 for 1937, part G.
[a]Percentages may not sum to 100 due to rounding.

Portents of Reform

In the depression, public debate over government health insurance did reach important milestones in three provinces—Alberta, British Columbia, and Saskatchewan—even if no programmatic changes instantly came out of those deliberations. Even though the crisis in government finance ultimately frustrated bold advances for compulsory health insurance, these provinces would later emerge as strongholds of public hospital insurance in the immediate postwar era. Alberta, British Columbia, and Saskatchewan subsequently formed the nucleus of a provincial coalition bent on securing an accord with federal legislators on national hospital insurance in the 1950s.

Alberta. Momentum for compulsory health insurance on a province-wide basis gathered steam in the one province where public hospital insurance had already established a foothold. Since the close of World War I, the Alberta legislature had prodded local governments to initiate hospital benefit plans in tandem with the formation of union hospital districts, the special-purpose cooperatives empowered to raise funds from adjoining municipalities to construct and maintain rural hospitals (Alberta 1922, c. 116). By 1930, approximately one-half of Alberta's rural population had obtained hospital insurance under municipal sponsorship (Alberta 1938, 282–83). In 1935, the United Farmers government passed legislation to extend public health insurance to all municipal districts as recommended by a special legislative commission (Alberta Legislative Commission on Medical and Health Services 1934; Alberta 1935, c. 49). Soon thereafter, the United Farmers went down to defeat in a provincial election, depriving the health insurance bill of a popular mandate. The incoming Social Credit government opted not to compel greater participation in provincially sub-sidized, municipally administered hospital insurance during the depression but extended tax-supported hospital plans to all rural and semiurban districts after World War II. Three-quarters of provincial residents would eventually receive protection from the municipal hospital plans before the advent of national hospital insurance (see table 4.2).

Saskatchewan. As in Alberta, hospital care in Saskatchewan had become increasingly premised on the formation of union hospital districts after World War I (Saskatchewan 1920, c. 213). Unlike in Alberta, very few local governments afforded hospital insurance to their residents even though the municipalities and the district authorities were becoming the ascendant sponsors of rural hospital service. Facing widespread insol-vency, local governments not only abstained from progressive experiments in hospital insurance, they largely retreated from defraying the operating costs of their own hospitals. During the depression, the provincial government assumed nearly exclusive responsibility for hospital subsidies—a flat per-diem grant to public hospitals for all patients, paying and nonpaying alike (Saskatchewan 1920, c. 212; see table 4.1). In the 1930s, a broad consensus had emerged in Saskatchewan that hospital financing was best left to provincial effort. For the moment, local governments had proved incapable of carrying out such a colossal assignment. The Saskatchewan Hospital Association joined with the municipal associations to argue that the future of hospital economics was a task of social engineering requiring the larger capital and comprehensive administration of the provincial and federal governments (Taylor 1987, 74). However, the sitting Liberal government had little room for maneuver. The Saskatchewan economy was the most severely depressed in Canada. The added expense of public health insurance was too much to ask for a government drawing so much of its revenue from federal grants and loans (Canada Royal Commission on Dominion-Provincial Relations 1940a, 160–77). With the wartime economic recovery and the subsequent installation of a Cooperative Commonwealth Federation government, Saskatchewan would become the first province to enact universal hospital insurance in 1947 (Taylor 1987, 69–104).

British Columbia. Despite a narrow miss in Alberta and strong grassroots support for provincial health insurance in Saskatchewan, it was a royal commission summoned in British Columbia that foreshadowed the evolution of national deliberations over health insurance. British Columbia's Royal Commission on State Health Insurance and Maternity Benefits represented the first comprehensive inquiry into health care finance in Canada. The British Columbia Hospital Association went on record in favor of universal hospital insurance before the commission: "The Association would favour a scheme that embraces all of the people; not with any limitations either for salary or age, or anything of that kind" (British Columbia Royal Commission on State Health Insurance and Maternity Benefits 1929–30, 2:351). In its final report, the commission outlined several formats for a provincial health plan. The one thing held constant in each of these proposals was a dramatic increase in public funding for hospital care (British Columbia Royal Commission on State Health Insurance and Maternity Benefits 1932, 40–45). The commission reasoned that compulsory insurance for wage earners would release the public hospitals from making annual appeals to provincial and local governments to cover their operating deficits, even though hospital subsidies in British Columbia ranked among the most generous in the nation, normally comprising 40 percent of hospital income (British Columbia 1926–36). As for doctors, the British Columbia Medical Association entered into negotiations with the provincial government rather than categorically opposing public health insurance (Naylor 1986, 60–61). In the 1930s and 1940s, Canadian physicians were convinced of the inevitability of health insurance in one form or another, and mandatory insurance for wage earners was the preferred option.

It is essential to recapitulate the evolution of Canadian workers' compensation laws to account for the political aspirations of British Columbia doctors. As the first system of social insurance adopted in Canada, workers' compensation had a profound influence on the medical profession's outlook on health insurance. In 1914, the Province of Ontario formulated a legislative standard for the other provinces and the federal government (Canada Bureau of Statistics 1928, 745). In each province, a workers' compensation board administered the program. Payroll taxes levied against employers were commonly pooled with government subsidies into a consolidated health fund that prepaid hospital and medical benefits for injured workers. The boards granted insured workers free choice of doctor and hospital. The health funds compensated public hospitals on a per-diem rate for semiprivate accommodations and paid doctors on a fee-for-service basis according to an agreed upon percentage of the provincial medical associations' fee schedules. Workers' compensation boards guaranteed incomes for doctors on equitable terms and posed no evident challenge to professional sovereignty over clinical decision making.

Whereas Canadian medical associations discerned in workers' compensation a select model for health insurance, the contrary was true for U.S. physicians. State-mandated health insurance for injured workers generally came under the financial and administrative direction of business corporations and commercial insurance companies in the United States, and corporate management of health insurance often infringed upon the economic and clinical autonomy of physicians. In the 1930s, U.S. doctors first resisted the extension of health insurance—public or private—beyond the realm of workers' compensation. Blue Cross hospital insurance eventually demonstrated to U.S. medical associations the possibilities for arranging employer-financed health plans that reaffirmed professional sovereignty over medical care. The Blue Cross movement cleared away many of the obstacles to a working alliance between corporate interests and the medical profession, each set against compulsory health insurance, to construct a market-based alternative to publicly financed health benefits. As with U.S. practitioners, Canadian doctors initially feared that private insurance would invariably challenge fee-for-service practice and would draw too much premium income away from medical fees into costly administrative overhead. However, Canadian physicians' immediate experience with workers' compensation suggested that public insurance was eminently preferable to the uncertainties of private insurance. The government-sponsored plans had assured paying patients without threatening reform of medical practice and channeled insurance funds to doctors with a minimum of administrative waste. At the outset, Canadian medical associations favored health insurance for low- and middle-income wage earners under the singular administration of public agencies. They hoped that mandatory insurance would preempt the rise of private health plans and leave to the profession unmediated access to high-income patients (Naylor 1986, 47–52, 63–70, 99–102).

Whereas British Columbia hospitals gave unqualified support for a universal program, doctors would only sanction compulsory medical insurance if they prescribed the fiscal and administrative terms of the proposed scheme, and the British Columbia Medical Association (BCMA) was determined to oppose the government when its conditions were not met (Naylor 1986, 70–89). Mandatory enrollment was to apply to workers earning less than $2,800 per year, a figure lowered to $1,800 at the behest of the BCMA. Over 70 percent of wage earners would have obtained protection under this reduced income ceiling. From the vantage point of the provincial government, the exclusion of high-income workers from the plan deprived the insurance funds of the contributions needed to cross-subsidize the enrollment of the nonworking poor. Against the wishes of the BCMA, the Liberal government subsequently decided to absent public dependents from insurance coverage. In response, the BCMA executed a volte-face to lead the political opposition to the provincial health plan, also delaying action on hospital insurance. The breakdown in negotiations between the provincial government and the BCMA concerned financial details, not the principle of compulsory health insurance as such. The demise of the British Columbia initiative would not prevent the Canadian Medical Association from attempting to strike a similar bargain with the federal government over national health insurance in the 1940s. Nevertheless, the political embarrassment of soured relations with the medical profession lingered in the memory of British Columbia legislators. A Liberal-Conservative coalition government would later divorce consideration of hospital insurance from medical insurance to sidestep any further confrontations with organized medicine. In 1948, British Columbia became the second province to enact universal hospital insurance (British Columbia 1948, c. 28).

The Federal Impasse

With the collapse of the British Columbia plan, the provincial initiatives of the depression era had run their course. In the late 1930s, the open question was whether the federal government would become the ascendant locus of legislative efforts to bring hospital and medical care under the rubric of social insurance. The primary obstacle to federal intervention into health care finance was that the Canadian constitution assigned jurisdiction over social policy to the provinces. Before the 1930s, slight measures of federal-provincial cooperation had issued from grants-in-aid legislation, most notably federal cost sharing of means-tested, old-age pensions under provincial administration. Given the extenuating circumstances of the depression, federal legislators were alive to the importance of radical social legislation. Provincial-municipal relief efforts had proven inadequate across the nation. Further, the hardest-hit provinces were the least able to raise funds for cash assistance. Only the federal government could restore the fortunes of the most distressed regions. Ottawa came to the aid of the provinces, absorbing about one-half of the cost of the relief effort and in the case of the western provinces over 70 percent (Canada Royal Commission on Dominion-Provincial Relations 1940a, 160–77). The superior taxing power of the Dominion, added to its much better position to resort to deficit financing, suggested that the federal government assume direct responsibility for guaranteeing a social minimum.

The British Unemployment Assistance Act and the U.S. Social Security Act did not go unnoticed in Canada and, indeed, could not be safely ignored. The sitting Conservative government attempted to establish a precedent for federal initiative in the realm of social insurance when it passed the Employment and Social Insurance Act (ESIA). The ESIA made provisions for the creation of a Social Insurance Commission to administer unemployment insurance and, pending further authorization, pension benefits and health insurance. The ESIA was never enforced. The Conservatives went down to defeat in the national election called shortly after the legislation was proclaimed, and later the courts eliminated all uncertainty regarding federal prerogative when they declared the ESIA unconstitutional. Judicial constructions of provincial sovereignty over "property and civil rights" barred the federal government from establishing social insurance programs without a constitutional amendment (Canada Royal Commission on Dominion-Provincial Relations 1940a, 247–49). As it stood, the Canadian constitution omitted any reference to an amending formula. The unwritten convention was that of unanimous consent. The federal and provincial governments would all have to agree to any concessions, and new grants of federal authority carved out of the eminent jurisdictions of the provinces were not easy to obtain. Health insurance was not likely to come under the direct purview of the federal government any time soon, if at all. The courts had acknowledged Ottawa's power to enact grants-in-aid legislation touching upon policy domains under provincial control. Thus, any movement toward a nationwide system of health insurance would likely appear in the guise of federal grants for provincially administered health plans.

Health care finance, in any case, was not the leading concern for federal legislators. The more compelling interest was to arrive at a national standard for income-maintenance policies. In Canada, there was no federally coordinated relief effort comparable to the U.S. New Deal. The Dominion's twofold commitment to uphold the constitutional prerogatives of the provinces and to keep them solvent took the form of temporary grants-in-aid of cash assistance programs under provincial-municipal direction. There was no shortage of criticism surrounding these legislative expedients coming from Ottawa disparaging the lack of federal supervision over what was perceived to be an inscrutable and haphazard assortment of relief-giving agencies operating within provincial boundaries. There were no other solutions to the problem in the time available, so the federal government opted to study the question further. In 1937, Ottawa convened the Royal Commission on Dominion-Provincial Relations to make recommendations for constitutional and legislative reforms. The commission offered a sweeping indictment of federal grants-in-aid of provincial efforts to address the emergencies of the depression. Correspondingly, it expressed a strong preference for dividing, to the greatest possible extent, responsibilities for social welfare between federal and provincial governments rather than encourage any further experimentation with cooperative ventures. To that end, the commission made an appeal for a constitutional amendment permitting the Dominion to establish national programs for unemployment insurance and old-age pensions. The other branches of the Canadian welfare establishment would ostensibly remain under the singular jurisdiction of the provinces (Canada Royal Commission on Dominion-Provincial Relations 1940b, 15–44). The commission neither demonstrated a thorough appreciation of provincial health policies nor contemplated a bolder federal presence in health care finance. In 1940, the provinces collectively approved a constitutional amendment giving Ottawa a limited mandate to start a national unemployment insurance scheme, but no larger consensus on social reform was in evidence. By this time, mobilization for war had alleviated the economic distress and thrown up other, more pressing questions of policy. Any further consideration of health reform was indefinitely postponed.

The Emergence of Private Hospital Insurance

Amid the crisis in provincial finance and the constitutional impasse over federal legislative initiatives, the provincial hospital associations began to explore the revenue-generating potential of voluntary insurance. In this endeavor, Canadian hospitals benefited from their privileged affiliation with the U.S. hospital establishment. In the United States, voluntary hospitals had already registered slight advances for employment-based insurance with the proliferation of hospital-controlled Blue Cross plans during the 1930s. Even though the disparate logics of U.S. and Canadian hospital policy would ultimately impress separate trajectories on health reform in each country, voluntary hospitals were the dominant institutions in both hospital systems and begat a sense of camaraderie among them. Canadian hospital superintendents often frequented U.S. conferences and developed shared outlooks on the technological and administrative dimensions of hospital modernization with their colleagues in the United States. Voluntary hospitals, U.S. and Canadian, faced a similar dilemma: operating expenses were mounting while revenues from paying patients stagnated. Many Canadians had also moved into the governing circles of the American Hospital Association, the Catholic Hospital Association of the United States and Canada, the American College of Surgeons (ACS), and the American College of Hospital Administrators. In the 1920s and 1930s, three Canadians served as presidents of the American Hospital Association: Malcolm MacEachern, George Stephens, and Harvey Agnew. MacEachern became the chief organizer and publicist for the hospital standardization program of the ACS. Under his auspices, ACS hospital accreditation became the norm across the United States and Canada. From 1931 to 1950, Agnew held the post of executive director for the Canadian Hospital Council (CHC). The CHC became the national umbrella organization for Canada's provincial and regional hospital associations and would later represent the hospital industry in wartime deliberations over federally sponsored health insurance. It was Stephens who moved to the forefront of the Blue Cross movement in Canada. In 1939, Stephens led the effort to establish Canada's first official Blue Cross plan in the Province of Manitoba. He later replicated this success in the Province of Quebec, and during his tenure as president of the CHC from 1939 to 1945, Blue Cross plans emerged in every province except for Saskatchewan (Agnew 1974, 32–39, 58–77, 155–64).

The 1930s marked the apogee of Canadian participation in U.S. hospital associations and the point of its incipient erosion as national debates over health insurance approached critical junctures in each country. The Catholic Hospital Council of Canada split off from the Catholic Hospital Association of the United States and Canada over ideological differences in the late 1930s. Soon after that, the Canadian Hospital Council faced the imperative of putting together a statement of policy concerning federal intervention into hospital finance. The immediate demands of political advocacy drove a wedge between U.S. and Canadian hospital leadership, and the fault line was no less apparent in the ideological loadings of the Blue Cross movement.

In the United States, there was some initial uncertainty regarding the political significance of voluntary insurance. Two opposing interpretations of the prospective role of government in health care finance accompanied the inception of hospital plans under the management of regional coalitions of voluntary hospitals. One account was that the emergence of these hospital schemes represented a transitional stage in the evolution of health insurance. Group enrollment for wage earners in Blue Cross prefigured the extension of prepaid hospital care to all Americans under a federal mandate. The other version was that Blue Cross represented a permanent foundation for privately financed alternatives to compulsory hospital insurance. The equivocation lasted very briefly. By the late 1930s, the latter interpretation had become the reigning orthodoxy for all three national hospital associations—the American Hospital Association, the Catholic Hospital Association, and the Protestant Hospital Association. Blue Cross would not be a bridge to universal hospital insurance.

In Canada, deploying Blue Cross as the principal weapon in an uncompromising struggle against national health insurance was not the pronounced motive of hospital politics. The importation of Blue Cross coincided with a sudden transformation of national deliberations over health reform. Notwithstanding the exhortations of the Royal Commission on Dominion-Provincial Relations to leave undisturbed provincial control over health policy, the federal government assembled a wartime planning committee to draw up a prospectus for national health insurance in cooperation with delegates of the Canadian health care establishment. In those collaborations, the guiding assumption was that publicly financed and administered health insurance would cover the great majority of Canadians. Private hospital insurance would supplement the government health plans. It was not until the late 1940s—after the first concerted attempt at national health reform had faltered—that the provincial hospital associations began to contemplate a future for Blue Cross as a vehicle for broad-based coverage. In Canada, the Blue Cross movement was a consequence, not a cause, of legislative paralysis. Government inaction, whether attributed to fiscal crises or to constitutional impediments, inadvertently prolonged the hospitals' recourse to voluntary insurance.

The differing legal warrants of U.S. and Canadian hospital enterprises channeled politics in opposing directions. In each country, antecedent hospital policy mediated the efforts of the hospital lobbies to discover and articulate standards for evaluating the appropriateness of legislative initiatives to reconstruct publicly financed hospital care. In the United States, past experience supplied the basic materials for constructing a vision of a reformed hospital economy that granted very little credence to national health insurance. Municipal sovereignty over hospital policy had privileged the creation of two functionally differentiated and self-governing hospital establishments—one public and reserved for the poor and the other private and mostly attending to patients of means. The defining maxim of the pre-depression hospital order was that of division, the partitioning of the hospital economy into distinctively public and private spheres. Extrapolating from these historical arrangements, U.S. hospital lobbies formed an image of health insurance that reaffirmed the classical segregation of hospital finance—government funding for the poor and private funding for the self-supporting. The national hospital associations uniquely identified employment-based, private health insurance as the medium for renewing the commercial foundations of the voluntary hospital system. Publicly financed and administered health insurance for the gainfully employed would violate the time-honored canons of hospital finance and would invalidate parochial sponsorship of hospital endeavors. As the argument went, national health insurance would precipitate government ownership of the entire hospital industry. The issue of universal access placed a distant second to the paramount concern over reinventing the division of labor between public and private financing within the emerging economy of hospital insurance.

The Canadian Hospital Council and the Catholic Hospital Council of Canada never subscribed to the notion that universal and compulsory health insurance was fundamentally incompatible with safeguarding the preeminence of voluntary institutions within Canada's public hospital system. Whereas public spending on hospital charity in the United States primarily abetted the construction and maintenance of local-government hospitals for the poor, Canadian statutes had manifested a long-standing bias in favor of nongovernmental ownership of local hospitals. Proposals for enlarging the scale and scope of public financing did not inspire among Canadian voluntary hospitals the sense of alarm with which U.S. voluntary hospitals beheld the specter of national health insurance. Since U.S. constitutions and legislators had demonstrated a consistent preference for investing in government-owned institutions, the political arms of the voluntary hospital establishment were unambiguously opposed to expanding democratic control over hospital finance. In Canada, universal access to hospital care had emerged as the corollary of making voluntary institutions the chief beneficiaries of tax-supported hospital care. The provincial subsidy laws gave equal priority to universalism and voluntarism and recognized them as complementary, not conflicting, elements of hospital service. The benefits of federal-provincial sovereignty over hospital insurance—in particular, the unique capacity of these governments to achieve universal coverage—were not understood as negating the virtues of local sovereignty over hospital management, voluntary or municipal.

Wartime Planning and the Miscarriage of National Health Insurance

In the 1940s, the federal government reproduced the Province of British Columbia's earlier failure to institutionalize compulsory health insurance. The collapse of national health reform had more tangled origins than the British Columbia episode. Ottawa was initially prepared to accept the key demands of the medical and hospital lobbies bearing on the financing and administration of federally sponsored health insurance. The Liberal government subsequently decided against legislating grants-in-aid of the provinces to establish publicly financed and administered health plans. Rather, the Liberal government submitted its health insurance proposals for provincial ratification at the 1945 Dominion-Provincial Conference on Postwar Reconstruction. The provinces of Ontario and Quebec jointly vetoed the federal offer for reasons unrelated to the specific merits of compulsory health insurance. The fiscal terms proved unacceptable to Canada's two largest provinces. In the wake of the Conference on Postwar Reconstruction, the fate of health insurance came to rest with the provinces. On the eve of the conference, the Liberal party had sought and won a popular mandate to enact national health insurance with the consent of the provincial governments. If the provinces demonstrated a collective resolve to reopen negotiations over health insurance, the Liberal government would not refuse them. In the 1950s, the prospect of obtaining federal assistance for tax-supported health insurance would eventually prove to be one of the catalysts for the formation of a provincial coalition seeking a national accord on public hospital insurance.

The Advisory Committee on Health Insurance

In the 1930s and early 1940s, Dominion-provincial conferences were not the only venues for intergovernmental consultation on health policy. And, the compounded difficulties of managing the relief effort precluded any sustained focus on health reform in those assemblages. A second, evidently more effective channel for intergovernmental deliberation on health policy existed, even if lacking the influence of more publicized forums. In the 1920s, the Dominion Council of Health was established following the introduction of federal grants-in-aid of the provinces for public health initiatives. The membership of the council consisted of the deputy minister for the Department of Pensions and National Health, the deputy ministers of the provincial departments of health, and assorted representatives of farm, labor, and women's associations (Naylor 1986, 98). In 1932, the Dominion Council of Health first considered the matter of health insurance. It subsequently passed a resolution calling upon the Department of Pensions and National Health to undertake a comprehensive study of the Canadian health care system with a view to laying the groundwork for anticipated negotiations over federally sponsored health insurance. In 1935, the sitting Conservative government opted to lodge this responsibility with the proposed Social Insurance Commission under the provisions of the discredited Employment and Social Insurance Act. Consideration of health insurance then fell to the Royal Commission on Dominion-Provincial Relations, which made no substantive recommendations for a national health policy. Undeterred, the Dominion Council of Health resurrected the issue in the presence of delegations from the Canadian Medical Association (CMA) and the Canadian Hospital Council (CHC) during World War II.

In 1941, the federal government received the blessing of the Dominion Council of Health, the CMA, and the CHC to draft a national health plan. In 1942, the Liberal government responded with the formation of the Advisory Committee on Health Insurance (Canada Advisory Committee on Health Insurance 1943, 68–70). The advisory committee was charged with drawing up a blueprint for national health insurance in cooperation with the national associations representing various branches of the Canadian health care establishment. By the end of 1942, the committee had fulfilled its mandate. It submitted for cabinet approval a final report that entailed a draft of national legislation authorizing grants-in-aid of the provincial governments to establish health insurance plans. The final report also included a model legislative act for the provincial governments to bring them in compliance with the requirements of the proposed federal legislation (Canada Advisory Committee on Health Insurance 1943, 3–43). That the committee made impressive strides in so little time betrayed the degree to which federal officials had cultivated the sympathies of the CMA, and the report faithfully adhered to CMA guidelines for health insurance.

Medical Politics. The CMA wanted national and provincial legislation that afforded a maximum of professional control over the financing and administration of public health insurance. Despite some initial vacillations, the CMA came to stress three conditions of the medical profession's participation in a national health plan (Naylor 1986, 99–107). The first concerned the funding of the provincial health plans. The medical profession stipulated contributory financing of health benefits. Payroll taxes on wage earners and direct taxes on the incomes of the self-employed would form the insurance premiums of the working population. In addition to these levies, federal and provincial governments would jointly finance the premiums for the nonworking population. The CMA wished to avoid a plan entirely credited against general tax revenues since, in its estimation, the provincial health funds would have to compete with other government programs for scarce resources. Establishing a separate fiscal system for health insurance apart from consolidated provincial budgets, akin to the financing of workers' compensation benefits, was perceived to offer the best protection from inadequate funding. Second, the CMA requested that provincial medical associations retain nominal control over the reimbursement schedules for medical services. And third, the CMA insisted that the provincial health plans fall under the administrative direction of independent, nonpolitical commissions. Ostensibly, members of the medical profession would form the majority on the governing boards of the insurance commissions. Appended to these superior qualifications was a range of lesser considerations described in exacting detail in the advisory committee's final report. They, too, revolved around legislative guarantees for private, fee-for-service practice and for profession self-government in the broadest sense.

Controversies about insured services and the extent of coverage were peripheral. Since the advisory committee observed CMA recommendations for preserving the clinical and economic autonomy of doctors, the scale and scope of compulsory health insurance did not trouble the medical profession. The advisory committee reported in favor of insuring a comprehensive range of medical services. The CMA had stated a preference for mandatory enrollment for those earning less than $2,400 per year (Naylor 1986, 108). The number of Canadians living below this income ceiling could not be estimated with total precision. Nonetheless, it was clear that no less than 80 percent of workers and their dependents would have obtained coverage under this proposed limit (Canada Advisory Committee on Health Insurance 1943, 477). Individuals receiving health benefits from the provincial plans would have risen sharply above 80 percent of the Canadian population once recipients of public assistance, unemployment insurance, and old-age pensions were added to the insurance rolls. In the end, the advisory committee reasoned that the provincial governments would have to make the final decisions about these eligibility requirements. For the purpose of estimating federal subsidies to the provincial health plans, the advisory committee assumed that mandatory insurance would cover all Canadians.

Hospital Politics. The health insurance committee of the Canadian Hospital Council was largely reconciled to the legislative ambitions of the

CMA (Canadian Hospital Council 1942). The principal clauses of the advisory committee's prospectus for compulsory medical insurance carried over into the realm of hospital insurance with only slight modification. One might wonder what relevance, if any, the elaborate legislative guarantees afforded to doctors had for the hospitals. The public hospitals had made large, uninterrupted claims upon the government purse since their inception, expected no less in the future, and had accepted all along public financing without any legal or administrative buffers to provincial supervision, which the CHC described as benign in any case. Whatever the arrangements for medical benefits, it was assumed that they could be made to work for hospital care. But the emphasis on federal regulation varied among doctors and hospitals. The CMA held provincial administration suspect and lobbied for exacting federal regulation of the provincial health plans. By contrast, the public hospitals tilted in favor of provincial autonomy. Too much federal control might disrupt existing patterns of accommodation among the provincial governments and the hospitals. This view was most pronounced in the thinking of the Catholic Hospital Council of Canada (CHCC). Since a great many Catholic hospitals were located in Quebec, the CHCC attributed an important role to that province in protecting the traditions of Catholic hospitaliers.

The disposition of the Catholic Hospital Council of Canada merits further attention. It bespeaks how differently Catholic hospitals constructed their interests in Canada and the United States. Among the U.S. hospital lobbies, the Catholic Hospital Association of the United States was the most dogmatic opponent of universal health insurance. National health insurance was socialized medicine. The Catholic Hospital Council of Canada advanced a much more forgiving interpretation of national health insurance. The CHCC unambiguously favored private efforts to enlarge the reach of prepaid hospital care. Yet, the CHCC acknowledged that employment-based hospital insurance was not a convincing answer to the problem, excluding as it did so many low-income workers, the unemployed, and the poor. The CHCC reasoned that mandatory hospital insurance was a practical necessity. If national health insurance respected the clinical autonomy of physicians and left Catholic hospitals under independent management, then it would not be socialized medicine (Catholic Hospital Council of Canada 1942). There was no comparable logic on the U.S. side (U.S. Subcommittee of the Committee on Labor and Public Welfare 1949, 503–16).

The Liberal government, rather than take immediate action on the advisory committee's recommendations, referred the proposals to a newly formed parliamentary committee on social security. In 1943, the cabinet charged the Special Committee on Social Security with reviewing the matter of health insurance along with concurrent initiatives to reform old-age pensions and unemployment insurance. In these hearings, the Canadian Hospital Council offered an appraisal of the public hospital system, interestingly enough, through pointed comparisons with the U.S. hospital industry. Though voluntary hospitals predominated in both countries, what distinguished Canadian voluntary hospitals was that they were *public* institutions. In the United States, voluntary hospitals were *private* institutions. The CHC prided Canadian hospitals on their commitment to the highest standards of service for all patients—irrespective of their financial status, race, or religion (Canadian Hospital Council 1943, 5–7). And while the council offered a positive assessment of provincial financing and supervision, it expressed a strong desire to relieve local governments of their obligations to subsidize public hospitals under existing provincial statutes. Public hospitals had grown tired of disagreements with the municipalities over reimbursements for the care of the poor. The CHC remarked that "trustees of hospitals . . . become discouraged over these controversies and would welcome an arrangement which would eliminate these sources of friction and anxiety" (Canadian Hospital Council 1943, 9). National health insurance, if implemented along the lines detailed in the advisory committee's report, represented an appropriate step in the evolution of hospital finance. The Special Committee on Social Security agreed. It endorsed the draft legislation and returned the proposals to the cabinet for further consideration.

In 1944, the prospects for federal action looked bright. The advisory committee had emerged from consultations with the Canadian Medical Association and the Canadian Hospital Council with an agreement on national health insurance. These proposals had survived the scrutiny of a parliamentary committee charged with bringing the debate over health insurance to the widest possible audience. Provincial ministers of health had declared their tentative support for the federal initiative (Canada 1945, 44). Much to the dismay of the CMA, the Liberal government opted to postpone enactment of the advisory committee's draft legislation. In the spring of 1945, the Liberal government dissolved Parliament. The CMA warily observed the issue of national health insurance converted into a plank in the Liberal government's reelection platform. The medical profession had made every effort to insulate consideration of national health reform from the crosscurrents of party politics. In the end, voters returned the Liberal party to government, and so the health insurance accords evidently survived the election without fundamental restatement. The

remaining hurdle was to secure endorsement of the provincial premiers—
a task reserved for a summit of first ministers. The next one, the Dominion-Provincial Conference on Postwar Reconstruction, would convene in late summer.

Even though national health insurance had obtained a popular mandate, the election introduced a new element of uncertainty into the political calculus of health reform. It soon became apparent that the provinces would not have the option of accepting or refusing federal assistance for health insurance on its own merits. The Liberal government had committed to comprehensive social reforms during the 1945 national election. Health reform became one component of a more ambitious scheme that included a prospective overhaul of unemployment insurance and of old-age pensions. The federal government melded the three initiatives into a unified social security package—the so-called Green Book proposals—unveiled before the provinces at the Conference on Postwar Reconstruction. A federal-provincial settlement on health insurance would come to depend upon a series of collateral agreements on these other reforms. Added to these complications was the overarching problem of reaching a consensus on apportioning tax revenues among the federal and provincial governments. In proposing to absorb most of the expense of a national system of social insurance, the Liberal government was no less determined to routinize federal sovereignty over provincial fiscal policy.

The Dominion-Provincial Conference on Postwar Reconstruction

In readying the Green Book proposals for the Conference, the Liberal government made two modifications that threatened the demise of the federal health initiative. The first of them was to forsake the requirement of uniform provincial legislation. The Liberals anticipated that the provinces would dismiss the financial and administrative provisions of the advisory committee's legislative blueprints as excessive federal regulation. The cabinet opted to limit negotiations to federal cost sharing and to leave to provincial discretion the ways and means of raising matching contributions to the health insurance funds. The provinces would also have a free hand in administering the health plans. While these amendments were intended to prevent negotiations from grinding to a halt over what promised to become points of serious contention, they called into question the medical profession's advocations. The safeguards written into the advisory committee's legislative drafts had formed the basis of CMA approval of the earlier versions of the federal health plan. These provisions had no legal status in the Green Book proposals. This tactic greatly diminished the medical lobby's enthusiasm for national health insurance (Naylor 1986, 131–34).

Setting aside the CMA request for uniform legislation may have lessened provincial objections to a national program, but this departure did not give every concession to provincial autonomy needed for an accord. Ottawa might have quickly reached a settlement with the provinces if the Dominion had devised a strategy for insulating the proposal from other, more controversial issues. This, the federal government did not do. The Liberal government made the Green Book proposals conditional upon the renewal of tax-sharing agreements. In wartime, Ottawa negotiated tax rental agreements with the provinces under which the federal government gained sole occupancy of specific tax fields, namely, income, corporate, and succession taxes. In return, the federal government extended per-capita subsidies to the provinces to meet their operating expenses. When the federal government insisted on prolonging these arrangements as part of an all-or-nothing deal that encompassed the federal health initiative, the delegations from Ontario and Quebec refused. It was this second strategy that frustrated any sustained deliberations over national health insurance. The conference ended without agreements of any kind.

The interesting divisions appeared not so much between Ottawa and the provinces as between the provinces themselves. Though intent on preserving their constitutional status, the provinces reached different conclusions about the federal proposals. The major provinces of Ontario and Quebec asserted their right to fiscal and legislative initiative apart from federal orchestration. By contrast, the minor provinces claimed that they could best fulfill their constitutional obligations if made privy to a greater portion of federal revenue. The former equated the right to tax with the right to govern, and so any prolonged concentration of fiscal power in Ottawa vitiated Canadian constitutional principles. For the latter, this principle was less obvious. Since the minor provinces looked to the federal government for financial strength, delegating their taxing powers to Ottawa did not necessarily imply any loss of autonomy if federal subsidies came closer to meeting their fiscal needs. In the end, the view of the two largest and politically important provinces prevailed.

The stated positions of Ontario and Quebec did not point to a lasting alliance against national health insurance. The Quebec government appealed to the unreconstructed doctrine of Canadian federalism in marshaling arguments against the Green Book proposals. The Quebec thesis was that Ottawa and the provinces had their respective legislative spheres clearly stated in the constitution and that each government should continue to labor in its own jurisdictions without encroaching upon the other's. Canada's fundamental law, went the argument, had reserved for Quebec the authority to protect the religion, language, and social institutions of the French-Canadian minority against the English-Canadian majority seated in the Dominion parliament. Provincial control over social policy was the intent of the architects of the Confederation, and so the federal government should leave well enough alone.

There was no parallel argument from the Ontario side. While Ontario governments have ardently defended provincial rights, historically they have not followed any course that ruled out evolutionary changes in Canadian federalism. It was the brinksmanship of the Green Book proposals to which Ontario objected, not to federal-provincial partnerships in social reform. As such, Ontario occupied the strategic middle ground between Quebec and the other provinces. As with the minor provinces, Ontario envisaged cooperative federal-provincial programs as the means for establishing a social minimum and acknowledged that this endeavor implied fiscal transfers from richer to poorer provinces. As with Quebec, Ontario was not prepared to allow the federal government to manipulate common interests in social policy to raise the Dominion above the political rank of the provinces. The Ontario government had no ideological quarrel with the formation of a national welfare state but was not willing to hand over a blank check to Ottawa. This populous and wealthy province reserved for itself the role of mediator of federal-provincial collaborations in the postwar era. Ontario would eventually arbitrate national hospital reform.

The National Health Program

The failed Conference on Postwar Reconstruction left the Liberal government badly divided on the matter of national health insurance (Martin 1985, 27–75). Public approval of a national health plan remained solid. The cooperation between federal officials and the health care lobbies manifested in the formative stages of the federal initiative, the hearings of the Special Committee on Social Security, the 1945 national election, and the declared aims of the Conference on Postwar Reconstruction had created long-standing expectations for publicly financed health benefits. As distinct from concurrent debates over national health reform in the United States, Canadians were not exposed to propaganda campaigns to discredit mandatory health insurance coming from the ranks of the health care establishment. Correspondingly, not one of the national political parties staked its popular appeal upon a declared hostility to universal health insurance in the 1940s and beyond, whereas in the United States, Republicans and southern Democrats bluntly opposed liberal Democrats' proposals for national health insurance. Nonetheless, given the fiscal and constitutional implications of health reform in Canada, public opinion did not necessarily bestow upon the federal government a mandate to proceed on its own. As an integrated set of propositions linking social insurance to federal taxing supremacy, the Green Book proposals had produced an impasse in federal-provincial relations. The Liberal government had no apparent intention of altering the financial terms of the 1945 offer. By mid-1947, the seven minor provinces had signed tax rental agreements upon which the social security initiatives had been premised, but the Liberal government refused to act on its blueprint for social reform until Ontario and Quebec joined the others.

The newly appointed minister of national health and welfare, Paul Martin, came away from the cabinet with a legislative compromise to keep alive the Liberal government's fading interest in national health insurance (Martin 1985, 45–54). Martin's plan for a nationwide program of accelerated investments in health care facilities had two simple advantages. First, it broke away federal grants to renew the infrastructure of the health care system from the fiscal terms of the Green Book proposals. Second, it omitted federal assistance for health insurance without betraying the Liberal government's mounting ambivalence toward federal interventions into health care finance. In May 1948, Prime Minister MacKenzie King announced the creation of a five-year National Health Program (NHP) to prepare the way for a delayed arrival of federally sponsored health insurance. The Green Book proposals had included subsidies for health care planning, public health measures, health insurance, and low-interest loans for hospital construction. The NHP left out funding for health insurance, converted the offer of loans for hospital construction into matching federal grants for the same, and expanded assistance for programs subsumed under the title of health planning and public health services. The NHP would ostensibly strengthen preventative health services and eliminate other bottlenecks, in particular, potential shortages of hospital beds and health personnel, which might complicate the introduction of national health insurance. The cabinet expected the NHP to appease the provinces that wanted immediate federal action on health reform, and with an election looming, the NHP might absolve the Liberal government of any political liabilities for temporizing on universal health insurance.

The connection between the NHP and national health insurance was much less understood than projected. Paul Martin received the blessing of retiring prime minister MacKenzie King to link the two publicly. The NHP received cabinet assent even though the declaration of intent to press forward with national health insurance only commanded the pronounced enthusiasm of King and Martin. It was left to King's successor, Louis St. Laurent, to make good on this claim. The incoming prime minister and the majority of cabinet ministers assigned a low priority to national health insurance among the competing demands on the federal budget. If voters could be counted upon to support health initiatives in the most general sense, and this was the prevailing opinion of the cabinet, then comparatively unambitious legislation would suffice. These political instincts proved correct. The Liberal government renewed its popular mandate in the 1949 national election. Nonetheless, MacKenzie King's proclamation had entered into the text of the Liberal platform. In principle, the Liberal government was still committed to national health insurance.

The Triumph of National Hospital Insurance

At the Conference on Postwar Reconstruction, the compounded jurisdictional disputes implicated in the sweeping transformation of the Canadian welfare state set back the cause of national health insurance because the machinery of intergovernmental consensus building could not bear the weight of the Green Book proposals. However, federal-provincial consultation and accommodation had not wholly evaporated. Progress was made when all the issues of common concern to federal and provincial legislators were not handled at the same time. In the late 1940s and early 1950s, Ottawa and the provinces concurred on significant amendments to unemployment insurance and old-age pensions. Working agreements on social reform could be had, in limited installments, when buffered from controversies over national fiscal policy. Incremental problem solving— narrowing the range of issues to manageable proportions at any one time—prevailed in the long term. The matter of publicly sponsored hospital insurance was settled no differently. In 1955, when a critical mass of provincial leaders stepped forward to press for federal grants-in-aid of hospital insurance, the Liberal government was drawn into fashioning a concrete proposal for hospital reform. After two years of deliberations over federal sponsorship of provincial hospital plans, the Canadian parliament unanimously passed the Hospital Insurance and Diagnostic Services Act in 1957. Under the national mandate, hospital benefits were to be made available to all Canadian residents on equal terms and conditions for all medically necessary in-patient services.

Breaking away Hospital from Medical Insurance

Soon after the Conference on Postwar Reconstruction, provincial initiatives started the country along the road to a national hospital policy. The provincial governments of Saskatchewan and British Columbia repealed their subsidy laws in favor of universal hospital insurance on a provincewide basis while the Province of Alberta greatly expanded the reach of its municipal hospital plans. These legislative advances gradually transformed the national debate over health insurance. Canada's westernmost provinces now represented a permanent constituency with a transparent stake in federal assistance for broad-based, tax-supported hospital insurance. Added to their ranks was the Province of Newfoundland. Before joining the Confederation in 1949, the Newfoundland government had assumed direct responsibility for the health care of its rural population through a network of provincially owned and financed hospitals. Collectively, these governments would serve as the principal counterweight to the withering allure of compulsory hospital insurance among the six provinces where employment-based health plans were becoming the dominant force in hospital finance.

The emergence of these strongholds for public hospital insurance foreshadowed the compartmentalization of national health reform. Until the late 1940s, reaching an accord with doctors on publicly financed and administered health insurance had obscured hospital reform as a distinctive realm of legislative action. Provincial legislators in British Columbia and Saskatchewan had discovered that their attempts to bring medical care under the rubric of compulsory health insurance had generated insuperable political turbulence. Efforts to initiate and to expand mandatory hospital insurance had not met with resistance when severed from medical insurance. Physicians had withdrawn their qualified endorsements of public medical insurance after observing the Liberal government's handling of the advisory committee's blueprint for a national health plan. The vicissitudes of party politics and of federal-provincial collaborations were now perceived as dismal foundations for medical insurance. Employer-financed and physician-controlled medical plans had become the heir apparent to the failed attempt at national health insurance. In the revised policy declarations of Canadian medical associations, voluntary insurance represented the most promising avenue for reaffirming professional sovereignty over the clinical and economic aspects of medical practice (Naylor 1986, 152–58). In the 1950s, there was little determination among federal and provincial legislators to explore the depths of this newfound antipathy to publicly administered medical insurance.

Forging a National Policy on Hospital Reform

In 1953, the National Health Program was approaching the end of its five-year term, and the Liberal government in Ottawa was also facing an impending federal election. Since MacKenzie King had unveiled the NHP as "the first stage in the development of a comprehensive health insurance plan for all Canadians," the Liberal party was forced to take a position on health reform during the political campaign. The government remained divided on the question of national health insurance. Prime Minister St. Laurent wanted to give maximum latitude to further investments in employer-financed health plans. Private insurer carriers had registered substantial enrollments throughout the duration of the NHP. To the thinking of the prime minister, if most workers eventually obtained voluntary protection, then the government would justifiably spare itself the considerable expense of arranging publicly financed health benefits for every Canadian. In cabinet, the majority still took the view of the prime minister on the financial implications of universal health insurance. Now that Canada was involved in the Korean War, military budgets had imposed austerity measures on domestic spending across the board. Most cabinet ministers feared that the proposed outlays for national health insurance, if combined with the heavy obligations of peacekeeping missions, would invariably starve their departments of badly needed revenue. Otherwise, the Liberal platform and the party caucus stood behind the government's leading advocate for national health insurance, the minister of national health and welfare, Paul Martin (Martin 1985, 219–29). The chosen way out of the deadlock was to refer the matter back to the provinces. Under their renewed mandate, the Liberals prolonged the life of the NHP as an intermediate policy but, more importantly, pledged to move forward with a national health plan when most of the provincial governments were ready to participate in a federal program (Taylor 1987, 205).

The *six-province rule* marked a significant turning point for deliberations over national health reform. First, other federal advances in the realm of social insurance—unemployment insurance and old-age pensions—had gone through with the general consent of the provinces. The Liberal government opened the door to launching a national program of enormous consequence without the explicit approval of four provinces and specifically against the will of the government of Quebec—the only provincial government resolutely opposed to federally sponsored health insurance. Second, a federal-provincial accord on health reform would no longer depend upon collateral agreements on other controversial measures. Many of the political frictions surrounding the defeat of national health insurance at the 1945 Conference on Postwar Reconstruction had diminished considerably or lost their vigor altogether. The spectacle of the Green Book proposals was not to be repeated. Third, the six-province rule distinctively altered the terrain of interest group politicking. In the 1940s, the first attempt at national health insurance gathered initial momentum from the acclaim of the health care federations. The current indication was that the provincial governments, and the provincial governments alone, would furnish Ottawa with legitimate grounds for proceeding. Of their own accord, the Liberals had preemptively removed the national lobbies from imminent negotiations over the design of tax-supported health benefits.

The fate of national reforms would now rest upon the balance of forces at the provincial level among legislators, hospital associations, medical fraternities, and other organizations with a direct stake in health care finance. These constellations privileged a federal-provincial settlement on hospital insurance. This was the reasoning of the minister of national health and welfare. Paul Martin had indefinitely abandoned his efforts to win cabinet approval for universal medical insurance. A federal program would have to develop in stages, with hospital insurance in the lead. Martin estimated that the hospital plans in Alberta, British Columbia, Newfoundland, and Saskatchewan were the only promising foundations for a provincial alliance of sufficient weight to break the opposition within the federal cabinet to health reform. To that end, Martin endeavored to orchestrate provincial agitation for national hospital insurance as the first phase of a comprehensive scheme and, in particular, to mobilize Ontario premier Leslie Frost (Martin 1985, 229–30).

The 1955 Federal-Provincial Conference. The Liberal government had called for the enlistment of six provinces to begin a nationwide scheme in the most obscure terms, generating demand for a clearly articulated statement of policy. The extended lease granted to the National Health Program left a mass of unresolved questions about the timing, scale, and scope of federal grants for health insurance. The NHP offered no timetable for releasing funds to the provinces, nor did it contain any agreed-upon protocols for financing and administering the provincial health plans. The equivocations of Prime Minister St. Laurent moved the Province of Ontario to the forefront of national leadership on health reform. As always, the characteristic instrument of provincial influence over national policy making was the federal-provincial conference. At the preliminary meeting of the 1955 conference, Ontario premier Frost insisted that the prime minister open discussions on government-sponsored health insurance with a view to clarifying the issues and to forging a consensus on a national plan (Ontario 1956, 10–11). The premiers of Alberta, British Columbia, Manitoba, and Saskatchewan concurred (Taylor 1987, 208–9). With the credibility of the Liberal government on the line, the St. Laurent cabinet relented, and health insurance was put on the agenda for deliberation. The motion from Ontario had changed the face of the national Liberal party. It discredited the notion that employment-based health plans would ultimately excuse the government for backsliding on universal health insurance. Premier Frost, a Progressive Conservative no less, had upstaged the governing party of Canada. The balance of power within the Liberal ranks now shifted to the proponents of national health insurance.

In January 1956, the Liberal government announced the details of its offer to the provinces. The Martin plan for national hospital insurance was carved out of a proposal that the Ontario government submitted for consideration at the 1955 federal-provincial conference. Premier Frost had appealed for federal grants to offset 60 percent of the expenses to the provincial governments for arranging in-patient care in general hospitals and for the upkeep of mental and tuberculosis hospitals. These federal contributions would also support home care programs to relieve the public hospitals of the burdens of convalescent care (Ontario 1956, 12–13). Paul Martin wrested from the cabinet a more limited mandate. The Martin plan assured a federal endowment for one-half of the national costs of providing standard ward care in Canada's public hospitals. The provinces were left with undivided responsibilities for funding mental and tuberculosis hospitals and for developing home care benefits. To qualify for federal subsidies, the provincial hospital plans were to guarantee coverage for all residents within their precincts. Added to this stipulation was an amendment to the six-province rule. The federal cabinet now insisted that the requisite endorsements for the Martin plan would have to come from a majority of provincial governments representing a majority of the Canadian population (Ontario 1956, 13–15).

The political and demographic composition of the provinces gave the deciding vote to the government of Ontario. Less than one-third of Canadians resided in the provinces holding a vested interest in federal assistance for publicly financed hospital insurance—Alberta, British Columbia, Newfoundland, and Saskatchewan (table 4.2). The Maritime provinces of New Brunswick, Nova Scotia, and Prince Edward Island occupied the least enviable position. There, enrollments in private hospital insurance lagged far behind the pace set in the Province of Ontario, but these provinces did not have abundant revenues to invest in comprehensive hospitalization programs. Theirs was the daunting fear of rapidly inflated hospital budgets, as observed in the western provinces, without any comparable tax base to underwrite the projected expense of universal coverage. British Columbia, Alberta, and Saskatchewan had emerged from the crucible of the depression as the first, third, and fourth wealthiest provinces respectively. Personal incomes in the Maritime provinces were significantly below the national average (table 4.3). These provinces housed such a small fraction of the population that if they joined ranks with the western governments the resulting alliance would neither represent a majority of Canadians nor flex the political muscle needed to win a more attractive financial settlement from the Liberal government. Whereas the Atlantic governments were prepared to accept national hospital insurance if political forces outside their control improved the terms of the federal plan, the Quebec government unconditionally opposed any further intervention into the constitutional jurisdictions of the provinces. Quebec premier Maurice Duplessis never wavered in his conviction that each province should work out its own solution to the riddle of hospital insurance independently of the others, apart from federal supervision. With nearly one-third of Canadians lodged in the Province of Ontario, a vote of confidence in the Martin plan from Premier Frost would satisfy the Liberal government's popular majority requirement. If the Ontario government refused the federal offer, national hospital insurance might be postponed indefinitely or irrevocably compromised.

Ontario Agrees to the Federal Plan

The dynamics of Ontario's electoral politics were not the primary motives for the Progressive Conservative government's interest in hospital reform. In the 1951 provincial election, the Progressive Conservatives won a lopsided majority without any clearly defined policy on health insurance,

TABLE 4.2.   Enrollment in Public and Voluntary Hospital Insurance, by Province, Canada, 1956

	Population (in thousands)	Public Hospital Insurance (%)	Voluntary Hospital Insurance (%)
Newfoundland	415	47	10
Prince Edward Island	99	—	23
Nova Scotia	695	—	27
New Brunswick	555	—	38
Quebec	4,628	—	38
Ontario	5,405	—	74
Manitoba	850	—	55
Saskatchewan	881	93	6
Alberta	1,123	75	31
British Columbia	1,399	96	7
Canada	16,050	16	45

Source: Data from Canada Department of National Health and Welfare 1958, 4–5, 23, 103, 95, 115.

Note: Canadian totals exclude Yukon and Northwest Territories.

whereas the badly routed opposition parties—the Liberals and the Cooperative Commonwealth Federation—had advertised their determination
to bring forward a universal program for hospital care (Graham 1990,
186–91, 235–37). Employer-financed hospital plans in Ontario had
reached the same milestones of those in the United States. By the mid-
1950s, over two-thirds of provincial residents had obtained private coverage, and the benefit expenditures of voluntary insurance comprised about
one-half of public hospital income (table 4.4). The extension of the Blue
Cross plans and commercial indemnity insurance to most Ontario workers
had blunted the appeal of compulsory hospital insurance or, at least, kept
it from becoming a salient issue for voters. What had moved hospital
reform onto the legislative agenda was the national Liberal party's insis-
tence that any federal measures primarily rested upon the initiative of the
provincial governments, and following that, the enactment of the Martin
plan for national hospital insurance virtually required the endorsement of
the Ontario government.

While the Progressive Conservatives had not faced compelling pressures from within the province to take up the matter of insurance reform,
they confronted no insurmountable political obstacles. Unlike their U.S.
counterparts, Canadian hospitals had not demonstrated any sustained

TABLE 4.3.   Income of Public Hospitals, by Province, Canada, 1957

	Public Hospital Beds (per thousand)	Hospital Revenue per Capita	Personal Income per Capita (1956)
Newfoundland	4.0	16	735
Prince Edward Island	6.6	16	768
Nova Scotia	4.7	16	999
New Brunswick	4.4	19	917
Quebec	5.1	20	1,172
Ontario	5.2	26	1,610
Manitoba	5.4	21	1,305
Saskatchewan	6.8	35	1,376
Alberta	6.4	30	1,418
British Columbia	5.3	29	1,618
Canada	5.3	24	1,365

Source: Canada Bureau of Statistics 1957, 20; Canada Bureau of Statistics 1958, 65;
Canada Department of National Heatlh and Welfare 1960, A32.

Note: Nonfederal, general, and allied specialty hospitals.

TABLE 4.4. Income of Public Hospitals, by Source and by Province, Canada, 1957

	Federal Government[a]	Provincial Government[b]	Municipal Government	Voluntary Insurance	Self-Pay Patients	Endowments and Gifts	Total
Newfoundland	0.3 (5)	4.1 (63)	—	0.6 (9)	1.4 (21)	0.2 (2)	6.6 (2)
Prince Edward Island	0.1 (9)	0.2 (15)	—	0.4 (24)	0.7 (48)	0.1 (4)	1.5 (>1)
Nova Scotia	0.2 (2)	1.0 (10)	1.0 (10)	3.3 (30)	4.8 (45)	0.4 (4)	10.8 (3)
New Brunswick	0.2 (2)	0.9 (9)	1.5 (15)	2.8 (26)	4.9 (46)	0.2 (2)	10.6 (3)
Quebec	0.6 (1)	21.1 (23)	1.0 (1)	20.5 (22)	41.7 (46)	6.9 (8)	91.8 (24)
Ontario	1.7 (1)	17.4 (13)	11.2 (8)	63.6 (46)	39.6 (29)	5.2 (4)	138.7 (36)
Manitoba	0.6 (3)	2.1 (12)	2.5 (14)	7.5 (42)	4.8 (27)	0.4 (2)	17.8 (5)
Saskatchewan	1.2 (4)	26.1 (85)	0.4 (1)	0.3 (1)	1.8 (6)	0.8 (3)	30.7 (8)
Alberta	1.5 (5)	12.3 (37)	10.1 (30)	2.7 (8)	6.1 (18)	0.6 (2)	33.5 (9)
British Columbia	0.2 (1)	33.8 (82)	0.6 (1)	0.5 (1)	4.7 (12)	1.4 (3)	41.1 (11)
Canada[c]	6.9 (2)	119.1 (31)	28.4 (7)	102.1 (27)	110.6 (29)	16.1 (4)	383.2 (100)

Source: Data from Canada Department of National Health and Welfare 1960, A32.
Note: In millions of dollars, of nonfederal, general, and allied specialty hospitals. Percentages are given in parentheses and may not sum to 100 due to rounding.
[a]Excludes federal grants for hospital construction.
[b]Includes payments from workers' compensation fund.
[c]Canadian totals include public hospitals in Yukon and Northwest Territories.

interest in forging an alliance with doctors and commercial insurers to steer public opinion against universal hospital insurance or to defeat legislative initiatives to extend publicly financed hospital benefits to the gainfully employed. The Blue Cross plans had not broken the social contract written into the subsidy laws of the six provinces that had opted to test the limits of employment-based hospital insurance. In Ontario specifically, the regulatory cornerstone of the Public Hospitals Act remained firmly in place: "No hospital receiving provincial aid shall refuse to admit as a patient any person who from sickness, disease or injury is need of treatment" (Ontario 1950, c. 307 § 11). Provincial statutes had neither abandoned the principle of universal access to hospital care nor abrogated government responsibility for the financial losses to the public hospitals stemming from their legal obligation to treat all patients, insured or uninsured. The Ontario Hospital Association (OHA) had no quarrel with universal hospital insurance. The appointment of three past presidents of the OHA to the Ontario Hospital Services Commission—the provincial agency charged with overseeing insurance reform—affirmed the OHA's willingness to cooperate with the government to bring a plan into operation (Taylor 1987, 146–50). The OHA initially pressed for one significant concession from Premier Frost. This was to designate the OHA-sponsored Blue Cross plan as a universal carrier for hospital insurance, in effect, to transform Blue Cross into a public utility operating under the superintendence of the provincial hospital commission. The OHA had no reservations about discharging commercial underwriters from the field of hospital insurance (Ontario Standing Committee on Health 1956, 112–14). The first indication from Premier Frost was that the government would honor this request. However, in making final preparations for the introduction of the Ontario hospital plan, the OHA and the government reached a settlement whereby most of the facilities and personnel of Blue Cross were transferred to the Ontario Hospital Services Commission. Under the new dispensation, Blue Cross regrouped to provide insurance for hospital amenities not covered under the mandatory plan, most notably the added premiums of obtaining semiprivate and private accommodations and private-duty nursing.

Canadian medical associations could not muster any convincing solidarity for or against universal hospital insurance (Naylor 1986, 156–57, 162–67). Notwithstanding their repudiation of government-financed and government-administered medical insurance, doctors had not expended any political capital to obstruct the initiation and expansion of public hospital insurance in the provinces of Alberta, British Columbia, and Saskatchewan. From a medical standpoint there was no overriding motive for opposing the government plans. The mandatory schemes had not crossed the divide between social insurance and socialized medicine. They had left the public hospitals under independent management and left undisturbed professional control over medical services within them. Improved diagnostic and surgical facilities in some previously undercapitalized hospitals evidently enhanced clinical freedom, and hospital bills and medical fees no longer represented competing claims on the incomes of patients. Nevertheless, Canadian medical associations had selective misgivings about national hospital insurance. They took exception to listing the services of hospital-based radiologists and clinical pathologists under the schedule of benefits eligible for federal cost sharing (Ontario Standing Committee on Health 1956, 89–108). Doctors wanted to establish a benchmark for publicly financed medical care whereby federal and provincial governments limited their efforts to subsidizing the enrollment of low-income groups in the Trans-Canada Medical Plans (TCMP)—the national consortium of physician-controlled service plans. Incorporating diagnostic services into a universal program for hospital care was viewed as setting a precedent for ensuing reforms of medical insurance that disregarded the profession's strongly held preference for means-tested government assistance to expand the subscriber base of the TCMP. Whereas the medical associations proposed separate arrangements for radiologists and pathologists, the hospital associations were equally determined that inpatient diagnostic services come under the jurisdiction of the provincial hospital plans. Federal and provincial legislators sided with the hospitals on this controversy. This led the medical profession to withhold its approval for national hospital insurance, but there was no resolve among doctors to mount any organized resistance to the implementation of the government plans.

The peculiarities of the Canadian insurance industry kept commercial underwriters from waging an effective campaign against national hospital insurance (Bell 1959). In the 1940s, Canadian life insurance companies had not envisaged a market for health insurance upon witnessing the medical and hospital lobbies negotiating the terms of a national health plan with the federal government. Canadian companies entered the market for employment-based health plans inadvertently and too slowly to acquire much of a vested interest in its continuance. U.S. concerns sold the great majority of commercial health insurance in Canada. Having misread political currents in the 1950s, U.S. insurers had not inspired the formation of a Canadian trade association akin to the Health Insurance Association of America, one of the enduring pillars of the triumphant opposition to national health insurance in the United States. Canadian companies were not willing to fight a holy war in defense of private hospital insurance given their diminutive share of the market. U.S. insurers could easily suffer the loss of their Canadian business since it represented only a tiny fraction of their North American premium income. Although the Progressive Conservatives more commonly gave sympathetic hearings to the legislative demands of business lobbies, Premier Frost summarily dismissed requests from insurance company executives to devise a government plan for those who could not afford prevailing market rates for voluntary coverage and for high-risk groups regularly disqualified from private insurance, most notably the aged and others afflicted with chronic illnesses (Ontario Standing Committee on Health 1956, 115–38, 153–88). The Ontario premier had no apparent interest in formulating a legal standard for dividing the population into two classes for insurance purposes: one of them entitled to publicly financed hospital benefits and consisting of those deemed too poor or too sick to obtain private coverage; and the other certified in good health and drawing sufficient incomes to arrange for market-based protection. To institutionalize this form of discrimination would require complicated, expensive, and time-consuming procedures and appeals that, in any case, would probably leave substantial gaps in coverage. With federal assistance for a universal program in sight, Premier Frost excluded from serious consideration arguments for a limited plan that put the government at risk of conducting routine inquiries into the health status and financial circumstances of Ontario residents.

Although the Progressive Conservatives were committed to universal hospital insurance, there remained two points of contention between the Ontario and federal governments that prolonged the legislative impasse in Ottawa (Ontario 1956; Taylor 1987, 150–51, 219). The first one concerned the matching contributions to the provincial hospital plans. Premier Frost still wanted a more generous financial settlement, specifically, to raise the federal share from 50 percent to 60 percent of the charges for acute-care hospital stays and to obtain equivalent federal outlays for mental and tuberculosis hospitals. The other notable exclusions from the federal cost-sharing proposals—the expense to the provinces of administering the insurance plans and of maintaining adequate capital investment in hospital facilities—also appeared on the Ontario government's list of fiscal grievances. The second controversy revolved around the administrative burdens of fulfilling the stated requirement for universal coverage. At issue was whether Ottawa would cofinance the provincial hospital plans from their inception even if they fell short of complete enrollments in the first years of operation or whether the provinces would confront the unenviable prospect of striving to comply with national standards without the immediate benefit of federal sponsorship. Premier Frost wanted assurances that federal subsidies would be made available to the provincial hospital plans at their commencement, allowing for a grace period during which the mandatory coverage provisions would come into force by carefully planned increments. Federal concessions on this matter would ease the administrative challenges facing the six provinces that had not yet initiated hospital insurance plans. This latter consideration ultimately held greater significance for the Ontario premier than his long-standing complaint with the federal cost-sharing arrangements. In March 1957, the Ontario and federal governments reached a compromise. Ontario agreed to the financial terms of the federal offer, and Ottawa agreed to fund the Ontario hospital plan from the outset if it covered no less than 85 percent of provincial residents. Subsequent to that, federal assistance would hinge on steadily rising enrollments (Martin 1985, 244–45).

Three weeks later, the Canadian parliament unanimously voted in favor of the Hospital Insurance and Diagnostic Services Act, the legislation authorizing federal grants-in-aid of the provincial governments to establish and maintain universal hospital plans. The governments of Alberta, British Columbia, Newfoundland, Ontario, and Saskatchewan had previously declared their intentions to participate in the federal program, and the government of Prince Edward Island joined them shortly thereafter. As required, six provinces representing a majority of the Canadian population had accepted the terms and conditions of the federal enabling act. The ensuing task of negotiating formal agreements with the provincial governments was punctuated by the federal election of June 1957. The Liberal government had gone down to defeat, and the Progressive Conservative party formed the new government. For the chosen prime minister, John Diefenbaker, the priority was to speed federal payments to the provincial hospital plans. The incoming government opted not to risk any further delays such as would accompany a thorough reexamination of the basic framework for universal hospital insurance already written into federal statute. In July 1958, the Progressive Conservatives initiated contributions to the hospital plans of Alberta, British Columbia, Manitoba, Newfoundland, and Saskatchewan in accordance with the provisions set out by the former government. As of 1961, the other five provinces had established programs eligible for federal assistance, bringing the entire nation across the threshold to social insurance for essential hospital services.

Conclusion

National hospital insurance resubstantiated the historical maxim of provincial hospital policy: universal access to the public hospital system. The winding path to federally sponsored hospital insurance began in the midst of World War II with the associated efforts of the health care lobbies and federal officials to devise a national health plan. The Liberal government folded these health insurance accords into a three-layered social insurance program—the Green Book proposals—submitted for provincial ratification at the 1945 Conference on Postwar Reconstruction. The subsequent failure of the Ontario, Quebec, and Canadian governments to reach a settlement on national fiscal policy stranded the Green Book proposals and fragmented the health insurance movement. Soon afterward, doctors rescinded their approval of compulsory medical insurance, opting to place their faith in voluntary medical plans. In Ottawa, the Liberal government stood committed to national health insurance in principle but offered no specific assurances to the provinces of federal action in the near term. As a result, the hospital insurance movement split into two branches. When faced with the uncertain prospects of obtaining federal assistance for publicly financed health benefits, most provinces gave temporary blessing to the advancement of employer-sponsored hospital plans. In four provinces, the tax-supported plans had become the dominant force in hospital finance. The Liberal government responded to the diversification of the health care economy with a vow to subsidize provincial health plans when a majority of provincial governments signaled their approval for a federal plan. Under these terms, the burden fell on the Ontario government to salvage progress on national health reform. It was the Province of Ontario that had constructed the basic framework of Canadian hospital policy in the prewar era, and it would complete the provincial alliance for a national mandate. Although possessing the most vital market for hospital insurance of any province, Ontario's singular capacity to invoke federal cost sharing of universal hospital insurance more than offset the political liabilities of abandoning employment-based coverage. Ontario premier Frost discovered, as had others before him, that health reform only became more negotiable the less it touched upon medical services. Rather than make one the enemy of the other, Premier Frost put first things first and set aside consideration of medical reform so that national hospital insurance might become a reality in Canada.

CHAPTER 5

Redividing the U.S. Hospital Economy

The Great Depression was the catalyst for reconstructing the political economy of the U.S. hospital system. As in Canada, the remaking of U.S. hospital policy represented an amalgam of three institutional forces: hospital reform, political reform, and historical precedent. The first generation of hospital policy was a matter of local jurisdiction. The determination of municipal reformers to sever the financing and administration of government-sponsored hospital care from the affairs of private hospitals had called into existence a two-tiered hospital industry and two hospital economies—a public hospital economy for the poor and a private hospital economy for the self-supporting. In this divided hospital establishment, the private institutions were the more vulnerable to business fluctuations. In the 1920s, the heavy burdens of hospital modernization had already shed doubt on the long-term viability of a private hospital economy held captive to user fees from patients, and the depression exacerbated the stringencies of individual budgeting for hospital expenses. The troubled state of the pay-patient trade created a unique opportunity for dismantling the historical segregation of public and private initiatives in the hospital field. For liberal reformers, the imperative of collectivizing liability for hospital bills pointed to unifying the hospital economy under the rubric of publicly financed and administered health insurance. The proponents of universal hospital insurance faced daunting rivals. In the 1930s, voluntary hospitals combined their energies to organize a private alternative to social insurance: hospital plans for the gainfully employed under the control of regional associations of nonprofit hospitals.

The transition to insurance-based reimbursement accompanied a transformation of the legislative frameworks for arbitrating hospital policy. Municipal sovereignty over publicly funded hospital care weathered the emergencies of the depression and World War II. Thereafter, it rapidly diminished. The local fisc had abruptly declined relative to that of federal and state governments. Before 1930, municipal taxes accounted for most government revenues in the United States. Washington achieved fiscal preeminence with the advent of the New Deal and the mobilization for war and, subsequently, became the chief locus of political contention over health reform. Federal legislators would ultimately take sole responsibility for devising standards for government-financed hospital insurance. Whereas provincial governments served as levers for national hospital insurance in Canada, without exception state legislatures issued the broadest possible warrants for the advancement of employer-financed, privately administered hospital plans for the working population. The political upheavals of the nineteenth and early twentieth centuries had divested state governments of any comprehensive interest in the financing and management of acute-care hospitals. In the postwar era, state governments assumed a novel presence in the realm of hospital finance as accessories to expanding markets for health insurance. In their new capacity as underwriters of health care for welfare recipients, state legislators presided over a marked contraction of the public hospital economy in the 1950s. The compounded inadequacies of state and local spending on hospital care for the poor eventually forced a national mandate for hospital reform.

Federal legislators observed the prevailing ethos of the first generation of hospital policy: the strict differentiation of public and private sovereignty over hospital finance. In large measure, the rise of congressional authority over government-funded hospital care validated the political agenda of the American Hospital Association, the Catholic Hospital Association, and the Protestant Hospital Association—the advocates for the nation's voluntary hospitals. The municipal hospitals that comprised the other branch of the prewar hospital establishment were not represented in national legislative forums. Preempting government-sponsored insurance for the working population was the overriding concern of the voluntary hospitals. In the 1930s, the American Hospital Association (AHA) surfaced as the coordinating body for hospital-controlled Blue Cross plans, the leading edge of the movement to renew the commercial foundations of the private hospital economy through employment-based insurance. The national hospital associations later closed ranks with the medical profession, various business coalitions, and the insurance industry to defeat national health insurance. In the United States, hospital reform would not become the portal to universal health insurance as it would in Canada. The other cardinal motive of hospital politics was to recast the public hospital economy. For the AHA, the depression marked the beginnings of a thirty-year struggle to routinize government subsidies to voluntary hospitals for the care of the poor. This sustained effort abetted the creation of two nationwide programs in the 1960s that leveled most of the institutional barriers to public spending on private hospital care: Medicare for old-age pensioners and Medicaid for those drawing incomes from means-tested public assistance. The new political economy of the U.S.

hospital system normalized government patronage for private institutions while reinstating the historical division of labor between public and private financing of hospital care.

Reconstructing the Private Hospital Economy

With the coming of the New Deal, the foundations of the U.S. hospital establishment—the separation of hospital endeavors into two noncompetitive and self-governing branches—appeared on the verge of collapse. Before the depression, public and private hospitals labored in their separate bailiwicks without encroaching on the other's domain. Municipal hospitals confined their services to the poor and obtained their budgets from local governments. Voluntary hospitals primarily attended to the gainfully employed and derived most of their income from fees. In the 1930s, the rapid ascent of federal tutelage over state and local policy making represented an implicit challenge to the historical entente between voluntary and municipal hospitals concerning their distinctive spheres of operation. If federal grants-in-aid of hospital construction continued to flow through state and local governments, and if the latter remained committed to investments in public hospitals as they had historically, the national hospital associations feared that voluntary institutions might forfeit their dominant position within the hospital industry. Further, the expanding public sector might jeopardize the solvency of voluntary hospitals if municipal hospitals increasingly attracted middle- and working-class patients—the acknowledged mainstay of the private hospital economy. These concerns had no analogue in Canada where government spending on hospital care overwhelmingly benefited voluntary institutions.

Against this background of looming federal intervention into the parochial realms of the U.S. hospital establishment, the AHA set out to articulate a political and economic program for safeguarding the preeminence of the voluntary sector and for reaffirming the defining maxim of the pre-depression hospital order—the partitioning of the hospital economy into two separate branches. It was an enterprise that implied two distinctive campaigns. One would be to reconstruct the public hospital economy for the poor. The other would be to reconstruct the private hospital economy for the self-supporting. As for the former, the AHA initiated a lengthy political offensive to reverse the spending priorities of federal, state, and local governments. Voluntary hospitals were now determined to break down U.S. legislators' historical preference for investing in government-owned hospitals. The AHA sought to privatize the public hospital economy by making voluntary hospitals the beneficiaries of government allowances for the hospital needs of the poor. However, the more pressing agenda for the AHA was to create novel sources of revenue to conserve voluntary hospitals' dominance over the pay-patient trade. In the early 1930s, the national and state hospital associations mustered their energies to reconstruct the private hospital economy through the medium of insurance. With their fees rising above the means of most wage earners, voluntary hospitals staked their future on prepaid hospital care plans for the self-supporting.

The Crisis in Hospital Finance

Michael Davis and Rufus Rorem introduced their landmark study in hospital economics, *The Crisis in Hospital Finance,* with this apocalyptic statement from AHA president Paul Fesler:

> Economic conditions on this continent and the rest of the world have seriously affected our hospitals. The decrease in bed occupancy, the increase in non-paying patients, the meeting of capital charges, the lessened income from private philanthropy and community funds— all these factors have added to the financial burdens of our institutions. Without being pessimistic as to the future, the American Hospital Association would be unmindful of the members' interests if it did not recognize the possible breakdown of the voluntary hospital system in America. (Davis and Rorem 1932, 3)

Notwithstanding the rhetoric of the times, the financial bind of voluntary hospitals had long been in the making. The depression hastened the final reckoning. The retreat of private philanthropy, shortages of paying patients, and persistent hospital vacancies had all become evident in the 1920s. Proceeds from endowments, donations, and organized fund-raising had earlier constituted a larger share of hospital income. In 1903, philanthropic sources exceeded one-quarter of all hospital revenue and accounted for over one-third of voluntary hospitals' income (U.S. Bureau of the Census 1905, 34–36). In 1922, these funds amounted to 17 percent of the receipts of acute-care hospitals and comprised 14 percent in 1935 (U.S. Bureau of the Census 1925, 4; see table 3.4). No sudden and massive collapse of charitable giving accompanied the depression. A cumulative deficit in private philanthropy, relative to hospital costs, had emerged over thirty years of expansion. And, the purposes of organized fund-raising had narrowed appreciably. By the 1920s, these proceeds were overwhelmingly pooled into capital budgets, not current operating accounts (Denison 1942, 26). In voluntary hospitals, capital investment in bed capacity, diagnostic equipment, and surgical theaters primarily benefited paying patients in private and semiprivate rooms (Davis and Rorem 1932, 106–23; Goldwater 1949, 65; Committee on the Costs of Medical Care 1932, 8). Much of this investment became tied up in idle beds. Occupancy of general hospitals approached 65 percent in 1927 and settled back to 60 percent in 1934 (American Medical Association 1928, 912; 1935, 1081). No drastic fall in utilization occurred during the depression. In voluntary hospitals, prolonged investment in private and semiprivate accommodations had engendered low occupancy rates throughout the 1920s. A 1929 survey of nineteen architects illustrated the changing pattern of hospital accommodations. Each architect reported the distribution of beds in hospital construction plans sampled at ten-year intervals (table 5.1).

The proliferation of vacant rooms in voluntary hospitals was a primary cause of low occupancy rates, as was the overabundance of hospitals in urban areas. Consequently, many hospitals did not survive the Darwinian selection of the early 1930s: 17 percent of government hospitals, 27 percent of voluntary hospitals, and 63 percent of for-profit hospitals (U.S. Interdepartmental Committee 1938, 45). Hospital insolvency did not greatly diminish aggregate hospital capacity nor bring down vacancy rates. Hospital failures prevailed among smaller institutions housing less than fifty beds and located in densely populated counties already generously stocked with hospitals (Mountin, Pennell, and Pearson 1938, 40–46).

These long-term, interrelated trends—the relative decline and changing uses of philanthropic funding, surplus private and semiprivate accommodations, and the concentration of hospitals in urban areas—had made for chronically low occupancy in voluntary hospitals. In the depression, the situation worsened somewhat as the need for low-cost and free hospital care increased. Although utilization rates only dropped about 5 percent, the distribution of hospital days shifted in favor of government-owned hospitals. In 1934, acute-care hospitals in the public sector were

TABLE 5.1.   Percentage of Planned Hospital Beds in Various Classes, United States, 1908, 1918, 1928

	1908	1918	1928
Large wards	28	15	7
Small wards	24	25	21
Semiprivate	10	25	23
Private	39	35	48

Source: Data from Carpenter 1930, 23–24.
Note: Percentages may not sum to 100 due to rounding.

running at 79 percent capacity, while occupancy slipped to 55 percent for voluntary hospitals. Government hospitals, including federal hospitals, accounted for 40 percent of all acute-care hospital days (American Medical Association 1935, 1081). And so, added to falling revenues and persistent bed vacancies came fears of incipient socialism. The desire to prevent government hospitals from dominating the industry became the controlling motive of the national hospital associations.

Finding paying patients to occupy private and semiprivate rooms was the understood method for reinvigorating the finances of voluntary hospitals. The fundamental problem was, therefore, a lack of purchasing power among wage earners. On average, white Americans consumed a little less than one hospital day per capita during the early years of the depression. But the incidence of hospital stays differed between social classes and between urban and rural residents. In the largest metropolitan areas, the poorest families received three times as much in-patient hospital care as middle-class and low-income families (Falk, Klem, and Sinai 1933, 115). City dwellers utilized hospitals more than those living in semiurban and rural areas, reflecting the urban concentration of hospitals and, in particular, of municipal hospitals for the poor. Hospital care for the wealthy and the poor did not preoccupy voluntary hospitals. The well-to-do possessed the means to pay directly for their hospital care in private institutions. The poor were the responsibility of local government. It was the otherwise self-supporting patient of "moderate means" that commanded the attention of the voluntary hospitals.

The CCMC. It was the "great mass of people of moderate means" agonized by escalating health care costs that the Committee on the Costs of Medical Care (CCMC) specifically had in mind when it came together in 1925 to plan an extensive five-year study of U.S. medical organization (Committee on the Costs of Medical Care 1928, 18). Funded by several private philanthropic foundations, the CCMC was an independent body of researchers drawn from a broad spectrum of health care professionals and academics: physicians, hospital administrators, medical economists, and public health specialists. In the early 1930s, the committee's final report brought the issue of health insurance into open debate. No discussion would be complete without examining the committee's conclusions since so much else was commentary on them and, for voluntary hospitals, an attempt to carry through with the committee's recommendations concerning hospital finance. The CCMC favored reorganizing solo medical practice into group practices based in and around community hospitals that would ostensibly fall under coordination of state and local governments. Even though the committee was not inclined to recommend any course of action that would indefinitely exclude a significant minority of the population from health insurance, it did not name publicly administered, compulsory insurance as the preferred vehicle for coverage. The chosen methods for paying hospital bills envisaged in the committee's final report were voluntary insurance for wage earners and government subsidies to private hospitals for the care of the poor (Committee on the Costs of Medical Care 1932, 120–34; Davis 1932). The CCMC emphasized evolutionary changes through private, collective efforts that would eventually reformulate the theory and practice of hospital financing so as to make them compatible with the achievement of universal health insurance.

Not all of the committee's recommendations stood an equal chance of becoming blueprints for the reconstruction of U.S. health care. The AMA opposed the committee on most every stance. Especially offensive to organized medicine was the proposal to form group medical practices within local hospitals. The hostility of the medical profession militated against any effort to reorganize hospital care along these lines. The accompanying suggestion of local and state planning of hospital care had no appeal for voluntary hospitals. The national hospital associations identified government responsibility for hospital care with the chronically ill and the sick poor. In their estimation, government regulation would debase the currency of private hospital care. Only if assured independence from public supervision would voluntary hospitals provide a beacon for the public hospitals to follow. Circumventing public regulation—as voluntary hospitals had largely done since the mid–nineteenth century—was a guiding principle of hospital politics in the 1930s and beyond.

It was the recommendations on hospital financing that the national hospital associations selectively appropriated from the CCMC: breaking new ground for private hospital insurance and obtaining public subsidies for voluntary hospitals to care for the poor. Both proposals held out the promise of addressing the problem of low occupancy in private hospitals. The AHA gave immediate priority to hospital insurance. Formulating recommendations for expanding government subsidies was the secondary concern. High vacancy rates of semiprivate and private rooms in voluntary hospitals troubled the AHA most. Reconstructing the private hospital economy had the first claim on the resources of the association. In 1933, the AHA ratified a resolution at its annual convention endorsing voluntary hospital insurance as the means "to offset the increasing demand for more radical and potentially dangerous forms of national and state medicine" (Falk 1936, 376). Rufus Rorem, who had worked with the CCMC, drew up the 1934 AHA guidelines for nonprofit hospital plans (Rorem 1934, 9–12). In 1937, Rorem organized the AHA Committee on Hospital Service, which began accrediting hospital plans as Blue Cross became the national and local namesake for the voluntary insurance movement. In the early 1940s, the AHA Committee on Hospital Service regrouped as the Blue Cross Commission—the national umbrella organization for hospital-controlled, nonprofit insurance plans throughout the country.

The Blue Cross Movement

The initiation of Blue Cross proved to be the catalyst for reforming and expanding employer-financed, privately administered hospital plans for the working population. Correspondingly, the voluntary insurance movement blocked the formation of a lasting, broad-based constituency within the voting public that would have otherwise sought refuge in government-financed and government-administered health plans. Blue Cross was not the first manifestation of privately administered health insurance in the United States; the widespread adoption of workers' compensation laws before the depression supplied the pretext for the appearance of employment-based health benefits. Workers' compensation laws commonly mandated employers to insure their workers against the cost of treating job-related injuries. Blue Cross plans strategically transformed the original contracts binding business corporations, insurance companies, hospitals, and physicians in the financing and administration of health benefits for workers. These modifications gradually dissolved the adversarial and conflict-ridden dealings between hospitals and doctors (as vendors of health services) and employers and commercial insurers (as organized purchasers of health services) that was so strikingly etched into the design of workers' compensation. Blue Cross marked the beginnings of a new era of mutual accommodation that foreshadowed the rapid expansion of private health insurance during World War II and that eventually cemented the political opposition to national health insurance.

Workers' Compensation. Under workers' compensation, state-mandated and privately administered health insurance violated three cardinal principles of medical practice espoused by U.S. medical societies: undivided professional sovereignty over clinical decision making; the right of patients to choose their attending physicians; and the asserted privilege of medical associations to determine the minimum fee schedule for doctors' services. In the great majority of states, workers' compensation laws gave employers the option of insuring their employees through a state agency, insuring through private insurance companies, or self-insurance. In a significant number of jurisdictions, businesses could forego health insurance altogether and take their chances in court. Most corporations fulfilled their legal obligations to arrange medical care for injured workers in one of two ways. Some hired their own doctors or contracted with a panel of doctors to provide medical care for job-related disabilities. Most businesses delegated these same functions to commercial insurers (Muntz 1949, 41–63). Employer selection of workers' compensation doctors lasted well into the postwar era. By 1949, only nine states allowed injured workers to choose their attending physicians (U.S. Department of Labor 1949, 8–27).

Corporate supervision of medical care was not limited to nominating doctors who were eligible to treat workers' compensation patients. Rather, it was integral to extending corporate control over medical fees and over clinical decision making. If workers had obtained the right to select their own doctors, employers and insurance companies would have largely surrendered their leverage in negotiations over medical bills. With this privilege going to corporate underwriters, they were able to exercise market power over individual physicians. Doctors competed against one another for access to insured patients and, thus, bid down their fees. Contracts for medical care under workers' compensation also afforded employers and insurance carriers the opportunity to exert influence, sometimes subtle, sometimes blunt, over clinical evaluations of the health status of covered workers. Employers and insurance companies had every incentive to manage their liabilities for cash assistance and medical benefits for injured workers by monitoring the clinical decisions of doctors and by pressuring them to certify patients as capable of returning to work. These arrangements for medical care carried over into the realm of hospital care. Hospitals commonly bid against one another to provide care to injured workers, and employers and insurance companies exposed contracting hospitals to various degrees of supervision.

U.S. doctors' experience with treating victims of industrial accidents sharply contrasted with that of Canadian doctors and impressed very different dynamics on health insurance debates in one country and another. In Canada, workers' compensation laws established publicly financed and administered health insurance for work-related injuries. Workers' compensation boards—the provincial agencies charged with overseeing the funds— made no allowance for employers or private insurance carriers to participate in the administration of health benefits. The boards singularly entered into collective negotiations with medical and hospital associations over the terms and conditions of health care afforded under the workers' compensation acts. These settlements preserved the workers' right to choose their attending doctors and hospitals, observed the customary independence of doctors and hospitals to determine appropriate standards of care, and upheld provincial medical associations' posted fee schedules. In the 1930s and early 1940s, these contractual arrangements became the inspiration for Canadian doctors' endorsement of publicly administered, compulsory health insurance for the general population. In the United States, workers' compensation converted the AMA into a vitriolic opponent of health insurance, whatever the financing—compulsory or voluntary—and however administered—publicly or privately. U.S. doctors initially resisted the spread of health insurance beyond workers' compensation, where it had disturbed patterns of medical practice considered acceptable to the profession (American Medical Association Bureau of Medical Economics 1933; Numbers 1982, 8; Starr 1982, 198–232, 257–74). The enduring hostility of the medical profession toward employer-financed and privately administered insurance did not suggest much promise for commercial underwriting as a long-term, viable alternative to national health insurance. In this respect, the Blue Cross plans played the key role in arbitrating the future of U.S. health care financing. The architects of Blue Cross consciously sought to vitiate the conflicting interests of employers, insurance carriers, and health care providers embedded in the operation of workers' compensation.

Voluntary Insurance. The cornerstone of Blue Cross hospital insurance was limited liability. Unlike health benefits afforded under workers' compensation, Blue Cross offered indemnity service contracts. Participating hospitals collectively assumed responsibility for providing a fixed number of hospital days per subscriber. Placing a clearly defined ceiling on prospective hospital benefits had mutually reinforcing logics. First, it excluded long-term illnesses from insurance coverage. Blue Cross plans had no pretense of integrating voluntary hospitals into the palliative realm of government-owned hospitals for chronic diseases. The primary objective of group insurance was to generate occupants for vacant semi-private and private beds in voluntary hospitals and, as such, to reserve for voluntary hospitals a monopoly over short-term, acute-care services for the relatively healthy segments of the working population. Second, the coverage exclusions of the Blue Cross plans made workers—as individual subscribers within group enrollment—risk-bearing parties. This, above all, proved to be the decisive moment in the evolution of private health insurance markets. In requiring patients to internalize the risks of paying for hospital stays beyond a preset limit, Blue Cross absolved employers of the imperative of regulating directly the fees and services of voluntary hospitals as so many companies had done under workers' compensation. The risks that workers now assumed were the risks that employers no longer had to assume. Blue Cross permitted business corporations to commute the variable financial risks of their employees' hospital stays into fixed premiums. Insurance companies were still laboring under the assumptions built into insurance contracts under workers' compensation: undivided liability for the potentially limitless hospital expenses of individual workers. To them, Blue Cross demonstrated the feasibility of underwriting hospital care through limited benefit packages. The unpredictable risks that workers now assumed created actuarially sound risks for insurance companies.

Transferring risk from employers, insurers, and voluntary hospitals to workers was the pivotal contribution of Blue Cross to institutionalizing passive corporate sponsorship of private hospital insurance. The hospital-controlled plans also departed from precedent in allowing workers to choose their attending hospitals and doctors. This was largely consistent with voluntary hospitals' efforts to institutionalize collective self-government through nonprofit insurance. Blue Cross plans operated on a statewide or regional basis. Subscribers were normally permitted access to any voluntary hospitals within their designated boundaries. Regional plans did not compete with one another, and they successfully prevented individual hospitals from organizing their own competing insurance plans. Patient choice became for voluntary hospitals the corroborating instrument of collective rate setting within the industry. Further, Blue Cross mollified doctors by reaffirming professional sovereignty over medical care provided within hospitals and by excluding medical benefits from insurance contracts. Blue Cross formalized a cooperative alliance between voluntary hospitals and doctors in the reconstruction of the private hospital economy (Starr 1982, 295–300; Stevens 1989, 182–93).

Even though business corporations and commercial insurers became integral to the expansion of private hospital insurance, and on terms broadly consistent with the principles of Blue Cross, voluntary hospitals initially carried a lingering suspicion of corporate participation in hospital insurance from their experience with the financing and administration of hospital benefits under workers' compensation. Many founders of the Blue Cross movement envisaged nonprofit, community hospital plans as a way to institutionalize group insurance for wage earners while circumventing employers and insurance companies altogether. The working premise was that employees would mostly subscribe to Blue Cross on a voluntary basis, that is, independently of employer sponsorship. Moreover, Blue Cross organizers badly underestimated the likelihood of competition from commercial insurers. Policies governing premium setting were based on the assumption that Blue Cross would achieve a near monopoly over hospital insurance. Blue Cross adopted community rating to determine the premiums for individual subscribers; each paid the same price. Community rating implicitly overlooked the possibility of competitors underbidding Blue Cross by cream skimming—offering premium discounts to lower-risk groups of workers. Given voluntary hospitals' incipient ambivalence about corporate involvement in hospital insurance, the national hospital associations were, as of yet, open to suggestions for obtaining government assistance to reinforce Blue Cross's emerging command over prepaid hospital care.

Compulsory Insurance. In the 1930s, the proliferation of regionally based, nonprofit hospital plans and the creation of a national supervisory body affiliated with the AHA did not necessarily rule out compulsory hospital insurance. At first, the exact relationship between the two remained indeterminate. The Committee on the Costs of Medical Care had likened voluntary insurance to an educational device that would ostensibly convince wage earners and the hospitals of the benefits of collectivizing individuals' financial risks of unforeseen hospital bills. Experimentation with voluntary insurance merely constituted a preparatory stage for government-mandated coverage. The grounds for this interpretation was solely based on the CCMC's observations of the historical evolution of European health policies. The committee underestimated the likelihood that shelving compulsory hospital insurance for an unspecified period might afford voluntary hospitals an opportunity to evade it altogether. Similarly, the CCMC offered no clues as to how long such provisional arrangements might last. Nor did the committee specify how voluntary insurance might be transfigured in the passage to a publicly coordinated, universal system. The national hospital associations had also not given much thought to compulsory hospital insurance. Although the AHA favored voluntary insurance as a bulwark against "radical and potentially dangerous forms of national and state medicine," the association never advanced any exacting definition of state medicine. The term originally denoted government-provided health services. But as the decade wore on, the AHA attached the label to any proposals for publicly administered health insurance. Even the expanding definition did not necessarily preclude hospitals from backing compulsory insurance that broadened the scope of the Blue Cross plans.

It first appeared that voluntary hospitals would go along with any federal proposals that expanded the embryonic operations of Blue Cross. This became apparent at the 1938 National Health Conference. President Roosevelt had intended to make the conference a forum for publicizing recommendations for a federal health initiative stemming from the deliberations of the Interdepartmental Committee to Coordinate Health and Welfare Activities. The interdepartmental committee consisted of a group of federal officials within the administration first charged with coordinating federally sponsored relief programs, but later it turned its attention to the problems of the nation's health care system. In a joint statement to the interdepartmental committee, the national hospital associations recorded their position as follows.

With reference to compulsory health insurance, our three associations have not yet reached a complete unanimity. To this much all
three associations would subscribe, that if provisions for compulsory
health insurance are to be understood as a prescription for every citizen to provide for some form of health and sickness security, all of us
would be in complete accord. In other words, if it were left to the individual citizen to adopt this or that form, provided he adopts a form of
economic protection in sickness, all of us would subscribe to such a
program. With reference to alternative plans, however, we might find
among ourselves some diversity of opinion. (reprinted in U.S. Senate
Committee on Education and Labor 1939, 647)

The AHA offered no clarification of this statement that betrayed an
awareness of the regulatory provisos that might cloak both voluntary hospitals and Blue Cross under a compulsory insurance law of this kind.
AHA president Robert Neff did not discuss this position when appearing
before the National Health Conference. Neff confined his remarks to the
troubled state of hospital finances without specifically proposing any legislative solutions and, further, did not claim to officially represent the
AHA in any case (U.S. Interdepartmental Committee 1938, 78–81). The
interdepartmental committee drafted its recommendations without any
clear understanding of what "diversity of opinion" existed among the hospitals. What the national hospital associations were prepared to accept in
a national health program remained unknown for the moment.

As the center of debate shifted from the National Health Conference
to specific legislative proposals, the AHA abandoned equivocal policy
statements and took a definitive stance against compulsory hospital insurance. In 1939, senate hearings on the Wagner bill provided the venue for
hospital spokespersons to hone their arguments against any federal plan
that trespassed on what they considered the sacrosanct domain of voluntary hospital insurance: the gainfully employed. New York senator Wagner introduced legislation authorizing federal grants-in-aid of state governments to establish publicly administered health insurance as part of a
larger initiative patterned after the interdepartmental committee's recommendations for a comprehensive national health program. Hospital testi-
mony before the Senate was mostly sidetracked by fears that the legislation
intended to create a government-owned hospital industry (U.S. Senate
Committee on Education and Labor 1939, 602–56). The national hospital
associations reiterated President Roosevelt's comments on the eve of the
National Health Conference that any national health program would
"alter to the least necessary extent the existing plan of cooperative understanding between public and private agencies" (U.S. Senate Committee on

Education and Labor 1939, 611). To the AHA, this statement implied that voluntary hospitals would remain the dominant institutions within the hospital industry and that Blue Cross would provide the foundations for hospital insurance in the United States. The Wagner bill had not premised the bill on a governmental takeover of voluntary hospitals, but the proposal did not explicitly compel state governments to designate voluntary hospitals and Blue Cross as the principal beneficiaries of mandatory insurance. The national hospital associations thought that they had reached an implicit agreement with the president and the interdepartmental committee to make voluntary hospitals and the Blue Cross plans the primary recipients of any government spending on hospital care.

When asked to choose between publicly administered hospital insurance and the nascent Blue Cross plans as the Wagner bill had asked, the national hospital associations indicated that they were prepared to sacrifice their proclaimed desire to see hospital insurance extended to the entire population if it implied abandoning nonprofit insurance as a bulwark against government sovereignty over hospital finance. AHA representative Claude Munger leveled an unguarded attack at the Wagner proposal: "We have stressed the belief that the care of the indigent and the medically indigent is the focal point of interest in the whole question [of publicly financed hospital insurance], yet the bill provides care for all classes. There seems to be no good reason why the government should furnish complete care for those who are able to pay for such care" (U.S. Senate Committee on Education and Labor 1939, 653). That the new era of Blue Cross insurance would confront the hospitals with many unpredictable adjustments went without question among the national hospital associations. It was also true that voluntary plans had not stabilized hospital revenues to any great degree in the 1930s and that their true promise remained uncertain. Nonetheless, the national hospital associations were unprepared for what they considered an extreme, unprecedented governmental presence in hospital affairs: public financing and supervision of hospital care for the working population.

The appearance of a federal health initiative under liberal Democratic sponsorship alarmed the national hospital associations. Voluntary hospitals had matured in an intensely myopic and parochial world. They had grown accustomed to diffident state governments. With few exceptions, voluntary hospitals had escaped state supervision to which the municipal hospitals were nominally exposed. And, state legislators had otherwise exempted them from minimal forms of public regulation applied to business concerns. Voluntary hospitals were satisfied with municipal activism as long as it was confined to providing hospital charity to the poor. It was their settled habit to think in terms of a monopoly over the pay-patient trade in hospital care for the self-supporting and of elastic commitments to the poor. The national hospital associations emerged from the worst years of the depression determined to protect these taken-for-granted immunities and privileges.

The Wagner bill ended once and for all the national hospital associations' brief flirtation with universal hospital insurance. Hospital representatives first argued that their quarrel with federal reformers was less in the realm of ultimate objectives than with the practical aspects of universal coverage. Willingness to consider a federal law mandating individuals to purchase hospital insurance—a transparent attempt to nourish the fledgling Blue Cross plans—had nonetheless suggested room for compromise. Taken to its logical conclusion, this proposal might have prepared the groundwork for transforming private insurance carriers into regulated public utilities. It was the first and only time that the national hospital associations put forward a proposal for universal hospital insurance. In linking compulsory insurance to public administration, the Wagner bill vitiated what voluntary hospitals perceived to be the middle ground of the debate over prepaid hospital care. The AHA stated without reservation that voluntary hospitals would have no commerce with government-controlled insurance. The association uniquely identified the expansion of voluntary insurance with the self-preservation of the voluntary hospital system. The basic thrusts of hospital politicking—private insurance for the self-supporting and publicly financed arrangements for the poor—remained wedded to the institutional motif of the pre-depression hospital order.

Proponents of national health insurance gained no assistance from state and local policies. Since historical experience conditions perceptions of future and uncertain realities, national health insurance appeared to voluntary hospitals in the guise of a hostile public takeover and of a condemnation of their businesslike élan. U.S. health insurance debates were not premised on long-standing patterns of constructive cooperation between public authorities and voluntary hospitals. Voluntary hospitals had primarily achieved their stature without assistance or supervision from state governments. Even though the national hospital associations came to idolize municipal control over publicly sponsored hospital care during the depression, the record of public-private ventures in the localities was far from idyllic. Local-government subsidies to voluntary hospitals began from a politically discredited past. Progressive reformers had done their best to eradicate local patronage of private hospitals. There were a few examples of productive arrangements between local governments and voluntary hospitals. The subsidy policy of New York City—as described earlier—was one of them. But these illustrations were not representative. More often, mutual distrust and skepticism tainted relations

between local authorities and voluntary hospitals whether or not municipal governments had made contractual arrangements with voluntary hospitals for the care of the poor.

The Canadian contrast could not have been more striking. Mutual
accommodation between provincial legislators and voluntary hospitals
had been the norm. By the 1930s, mandatory hospital subsidies had
acquired a long and dignified history. Provincial and local budgeting for
hospital care had protected voluntary institutions from deprivation
through the leanest years of the depression. The hospitals accepted the
right and obligation of provincial governments to guarantee universal
access to care, just as provinces expected local hospitals to retain maximum self-direction over their day-to-day operations. This was taken for
granted in health insurance debates. Canadian voluntary hospitals never
globalized the concept of institutional survival and autonomy to include
insurance arrangements. They expressed no unbridled fear of publicly
financed and administered hospital insurance as U.S. hospital associations
did. Public financing and regulation were integral to the dominance of voluntary institutions within Canada's public hospital system. In the United
States, public insurance and private hospital care became construed as
mutually exclusive in the imagination of the national hospital associations.

The Dilemma of Publicly Sponsored Hospital Care

If Blue Cross was the prospective medium for reconstructing the private
hospital economy, the open question was how the public hospital economy would assume its modern form. The major plank of the political platform handed to the AHA by the Committee on the Costs of Medical Care
was that governments liberalize subsidies to nonprofit hospitals for the
care of the poor. Even though employment-based, private insurance was
increasingly identified with preempting compulsory hospital insurance of
any kind, there were compelling reasons to pressure governments to
become "orderly" purchasers of care for a minority of the population. A
successful campaign for public subsidies promised to do away with
uncompensated care in voluntary hospitals and to reverse the uninterrupted expansion of the public hospital system. It is uncertain whether
public hospital capacity would have ever surpassed that of voluntary hospitals, but the AHA was not inclined to take any chances when the inadequacies of hospital care had become an object of national concern. The
formation of a two-tiered hospital system before the depression had
emerged from continuous investments in municipal hospitals. These
investments accelerated in the 1930s. During the depression, Congress did
not include subsidies for voluntary hospital construction in federally

assisted relief projects. Public works projects recapitalized government-owned hospitals. Between 1930 and 1940, the proportion of acute-care beds housed in nonfederal, public hospitals increased from 24 percent to 30 percent (American Medical Association 1941). To prevent demands for affordable hospital care from triggering further investments in the public institutions, the national hospital associations resolved that voluntary hospitals should work toward purchasing agreements with local authorities. The initial experience with federal relief efforts suggested to the AHA that Congress could not be trusted to engineer a program that would safeguard the dominance of voluntary hospitals.

It remained to be seen whether the AHA's newfound interest in seeking out cooperative financial agreements with municipalities would gain any assistance from the Canadian example. AHA leadership was schooled in Canadian hospital policy. In the 1930s, the AHA twice held its annual convention in Toronto as these meetings coincided with the appointment of Canadians to the presidency of the association. Harvey Agnew, the long-standing executive director of the Canadian Hospital Council, presided over the AHA during the second pilgrimage to Toronto in 1939. Throughout the depression, it was Agnew who endeavored to inform AHA planning committees of the modus operandi of Canadian subsidy laws. "What might the United States learn from Canada?" Agnew queried in a presentation at the 1935 AHA convention. In Canada, the uniform policy of compulsory provincial-municipal subsidies to voluntary hospitals, answered Agnew, had militated against the growth of government-owned hospitals and stabilized hospital budgets as evidenced in drastically lower rates of hospital closings in Canada relative to the United States. The Canadian experience might be of some value to the AHA as it considered proposals to expand government funding of voluntary hospitals, or so Agnew thought (Agnew 1935, 894–95).

S. S. Goldwater offered a telling response to Agnew's statements that suggested that the U.S. debate over hospital subsidies would have little to do with cross-the-border learning. In 1909, Goldwater had first familiarized himself with Canadian hospital policy in preparing a report on public subsidies for the AHA (Goldwater 1909). Twenty-five years later, Goldwater continued to praise Canadian methods. "Canada is paving the way to many hospital reforms," Goldwater started, "and particularly the relation between public and private authorities in the assistance of private hospitals. There has been far more pioneering and right thinking done by our Canadian friends than has been exhibited in this country." Nonetheless, U.S. conditions made the application of Canadian policies impossible: "I do not entirely agree that the uniformity of Canada's practice . . . is desirable in this country. I believe heartily in the principle of local self-direction in these matters. Not only should localities be free to introduce methods of their own, but that individual hospitals should be as far as possible left to their own autonomy with respect to their affairs" (Goldwater 1935, 909–10). For voluntary hospitals, municipal sovereignty over hospital policy was still the reigning orthodoxy during the depression.

In 1937, a joint committee of the American Hospital Association and the American Public Welfare Association (APWA) issued a general policy statement concerning subsidies to voluntary hospitals that reaffirmed local-government jurisdiction over publicly sponsored hospital care (American Hospital Association and American Public Welfare Association 1938). The committee avoided any suggestion of state-mandated subsidies to private hospitals. There were two central points of interest in the policy guidelines. First, the committee recommended substituting per-diem grants to voluntary hospitals for lump-sum subsidies. Under lump-sum arrangements, some hospitals had suffered financially for having taken on virtually unlimited charity obligations in return for a fixed annual payment. Other private hospitals had profited from lump-sum grants in the absence of adequate supervision over charitable services rendered. The committee also sought to end the practice of having voluntary hospitals bid against each other for the care of public charges. It recommended that hospitals organize themselves into local hospital councils to present a united front to the local authorities when negotiating subsidy agreements. The committee argued that municipal preferences for bargaining individually with private hospitals and for awarding contracts on a low-cost basis inhibited quality care. Second, the committee declared that public spending on hospital care should be confined to public institutions wherever the localities owned and operated their own hospitals. Public hospitals should have a preemptive claim on municipal budgets, and subsidies to private hospitals should never compete with local appropriations for municipal hospitals.

The AHA-APWA policy statement badly suffered from its own contradictory thrusts. On the one hand, it called for preserving the institutional basis of the pre-depression hospital order—separate, public hospitals for the poor and private hospitals for the self-supporting. On the other hand, it sought to discourage any future investments in public hospitals that might threaten the preeminence of voluntary hospitals. By one estimate, one-half of all cities operating their own hospitals also subsidized voluntary hospitals to a small degree (Agnew 1935, 892). The committee's suggestions, religiously observed, would have substantially diminished the number of private hospitals receiving public subsidies. The inconsistency went unqualified. There was another glaring problem with these policy proposals that made them appear like a halting and confused effort to grapple with the question of publicly sponsored hospital care: the importance accorded to municipal control over hospital policy. The notion that local governments could provide the material resources to observe the committee's recommendations betrayed a misunderstanding of how the U.S. system of government had changed during the depression. With the coming of the New Deal, the fiscal and programmatic aspects of local welfare policy were progressively falling under state mandates, which, in turn, were formulated in response to federal grants-in-aid of public assistance. Discretionary spending on hospital care ran into direct competition with statutory expenditures that the states had unloaded upon local governments. Federal grants-in-aid gave no priority to stimulating public spending on private hospital care. Until 1950, federal programs only reimbursed state governments for cash payments to recipients of public assistance. Beneficiaries were more often required to provide for their own health care out of their public assistance allowance. Not surprisingly, very little of this money found its way into the accounts of hospitals (White 1952b).

In the 1940s, the AHA would abandon its hope that the municipalities would, of their own accord, remain the public vehicle for observing the historical norms of hospital financing—strictly controlled, but adequate, government funding for the poor and unsupervised, private financing for the working population. In the depression, the AHA initially endeavored to prevent state and federal governments from becoming the loci of hospital reform. Unlike state and federal governments, the local authorities possessed neither the constitutional authority nor the fiscal resources to gain decisive leverage over hospital financing. After World War II, the national hospital associations reluctantly began to acknowledge that local sovereignty over hospital policy was crumbling. The AHA would find itself back on the doorstep of the federal government. This time, it would be to lobby for national policies aimed at reconstructing state and local hospital programs for the poor while opposing universal hospital insurance.

Hospital politics during the depression signaled trouble ahead for cooperative ventures between federal legislators and voluntary hospitals devoted to reforming publicly sponsored hospital care. Even though the Roosevelt administration had only made tentative inquiries into hospital finances without any firm commitment to a national health policy, there were already outward signs of two emerging political coalitions holding opposing visions of U.S. hospital insurance. In the minority, liberal Democrats in Congress and in the administration saw federally funded and state-administered insurance as the only promising basis for delivering hospital care to the entire population. It was difficult for them to see in the voluntary hospital plans and local relief efforts—unevenly distributed as they were and greatly varied in their legal and administrative arrangements—any hope of bringing hospital care within reach of all citizens who needed it. Even so, national hospital insurance could build upon the existing capacity of voluntary and municipal hospitals. Liberal reformers had not yet waged their final assaults on private insurance. And, they would endeavor to defeat legislative initiatives to expand the scope of voluntary insurance coverage. To this "public goods" conception of hospital care, the national hospital associations juxtaposed their own time-honored notions of local initiative, voluntarism, free enterprise, and independence from public regulation.

In the majority, Blue Cross was becoming a rallying point for the concerted opposition of Republicans and southern Democrats to publicly financed and administered health insurance. It was this conservative alliance with which the national hospital associations had first pooled their political capital. Whatever shortcomings voluntary insurance demonstrated in its earliest stages, the national hospital associations held that correcting these inadequacies only required time and that continued efforts to institutionalize employment-based coverage were justified. Not until the late 1950s—once private insurance had became thoroughly ensconced and liberal reformers had surrendered their campaign for national health insurance—would the AHA break ranks from the political coalition opposed to federal sovereignty over hospital policy. The AHA would then endeavor to build a coalition with liberal Democrats to reconstruct government-sponsored hospital care for recipients of income-maintenance programs.

Reconstructing the Public Hospital Economy

When Harry Truman succeeded the late Franklin D. Roosevelt in the spring of 1945, he abandoned his predecessor's cautious approach to health care reform. President Truman and liberal Democrats in Congress envisaged state governments as junior partners in a publicly financed and administered health insurance system under federal direction. Their proposals for universal health insurance would have afforded comprehensive coverage for all medically necessary health services. In the latter half of the 1940s, liberal Democrats set out to wage a losing war on two fronts. Southern Democrats and Republicans who steered congressional committees were jointly opposed to any further intervention into state jurisdictions. Beyond Congress, proposals for national health insurance faced the implacable hostility of the medical profession, voluntary hospitals, commercial and nonprofit insurance carriers, and assorted business lobbies (Poen 1979; Starr 1982, 280–89).

The American Hospital Association, the Catholic Hospital Association, the Protestant Hospital Association, and the Blue Cross Commission disparaged national health insurance as revolutionary and out of keeping with the historical evolution of hospital financing in the United States. The hospital lobbies claimed that the nation's voluntary hospitals afforded the most scientifically advanced care in the world and had achieved their stature with private financing, free of public regulation. National health insurance would rob voluntary hospitals of their raison d'être and would seriously undermine the quality of hospital care. The national hospital associations instructed federal legislators to leave undisturbed the efforts of voluntary hospitals, private insurers, employers, and workers to reconstruct the private hospital economy for the self-supporting. The singularly appropriate role for Congress was to assist the states and localities to honor these governments' limited mandate to provide for the poor (U.S. Senate Committee on Education and Labor 1946, 1689–1787; U.S. Senate Subcommittee of the Committee on Labor and Public Welfare 1949, 332–69, 405–16, 438–91, 503–16).

With the defeat of universal health insurance, two transformations in the U.S. welfare state created the pretext for federal initiatives to reconstruct the public hospital economy. The first had its origins in the Social Security Act. In the 1950s, congressional revisions of old-age pension eligibility made the federal government the principal benefactor of the aged. Before 1950, most elderly received income supports from means-tested old-age assistance programs under the immediate charge of state and local governments. The dramatic expansion of old-age insurance took the vast majority of the aged off public assistance rolls and made them direct beneficiaries of federally mandated social insurance. Political pressure for federal sovereignty over publicly sponsored hospital care first built up steam in response to the inadequacies of hospital insurance for the aged. The hospital needs of the elderly had become an object of constant concern in the 1950s and early 1960s. Dozens of government studies and privately arranged inquiries confirmed the commonly shared assumption that the aged required much more hospitalization than other public dependents. And, old-age pensioners confronted formidable barriers to securing individual policies from insurance markets anchored in employer-financed group coverage.

The rise of unmediated national responsibility for the well-being of the elderly contributed one part of the equation leading to federal dominance over publicly sponsored hospital care. The second impetus to federal intervention was the uninterrupted decay of municipal provisions for the poor in the 1950s and 1960s, without any offsetting investments in hospital care from state governments. The postwar advent of federal subsidies for hospital construction—combined with the steady expansion of private hospital insurance—recapitalized private hospitals to a much greater extent than public hospitals. The relative decline of municipal accommodations for the sick poor, and the attendant absorption of government hospitals into the commerce of insurance-based reimbursement, systematically implicated voluntary hospitals in the care of the uninsured. Consequently, the AHA and its insurance subsidiary, Blue Cross, became the leading advocates within the health care industry for congressional authority to restore public responsibility for financing the health care of public dependents.

Federal Funding, State Administration, Hospital Construction, and Local Sovereignty

Notwithstanding congressional opposition to national health insurance, federal legislators set important precedents for postwar hospital policy in connection with the mobilization. Congress had deep reserves of legislative resolve on matters directly related to national preparedness. Federal policies that would have otherwise become mired in controversy gained easy passage when established as military necessities. The 1941 Lanham Housing Act and the 1943 Emergency Maternity and Infant Care Program (EMIC) represented two such examples of legislative expediency (Stevens 1989, 208–11). The Lanham Act authorized federal subsidies for civilian hospital construction and other badly needed community services in rapidly growing populations near military bases and defense-related manufacturing centers. EMIC defrayed the costs of maternity and infant care for the wives and children of enlisted men. Under the provisions of Lanham and EMIC, government and voluntary institutions were for the first time placed on an equal footing in the allocation of public subsidies for civilian hospitals. State governments administered federal outlays to participating local hospitals that remained exempt from federal regulation. These were the precedents that would guide congressional policy making in the immediate postwar era. Federal subsidies, administered through the states, would bow to the local sovereigns of hospital enterprises, municipal and voluntary.

Lanham and EMIC were initially met with ambivalence from the national hospital associations. Although temporarily arranged and strictly circumscribed, these programs rekindled fears of unchecked federal sovereignty over voluntary hospitals. Washington had become the preeminent force in hospital planning with the introduction of Lanham. The United States Public Health Service (USPHS) supervised the hospital construction aspect of Lanham. The agency became the repository for expertise in conducting surveys, in estimating appropriate ratios of hospital beds to service populations, and in targeting public investments in construction as an integrated exercise. Under EMIC, federal administrators devised accounting methods for estimating the capital and operating costs of hospital services that were much more advanced than the rudimentary audits performed by the Blue Cross plans. Federal agencies had acquired much of the managerial and bookkeeping experience needed to implement national health insurance, if Congress so desired.

The Lanham Act was more disconcerting for the representatives of voluntary hospitals than EMIC. Even though EMIC created a working model for federally financed and state-administered hospital benefits that could be easily translated into a national program for hospital insurance, voluntary hospitals had already secured a beachhead with the Blue Cross plans from which they could wage the battle for control of hospital finance. Voluntary hospitals had no accompanying strengths in the field of hospital planning. The national hospital associations had neither applied any organizational resources to hospital planning nor reached any consensus among themselves that might have been brought to bear on congressional policy making. Though admitting that facilities were lacking in many regions, the AHA had not expended any energy on devising programmatic recommendations for hospital expansion, quite the contrary. In the late 1930s, the AHA had begun to organize an effort to reduce the nation's stock of hospital beds. The AHA had taken an inspired interest in promoting state licensing laws, driven by the motive of running out of business over two thousand hospitals—overwhelmingly for-profit enterprises—failing to meet AMA registration standards. As late as 1943, the AHA publicly declared itself in favor of extending federal grants-in-aid of hospital construction only if they benefited established voluntary and municipal hospitals (Hamilton 1943). The national hospital associations were still consumed by the notion that prolonged federal sponsorship of hospital construction would likely privilege the growth of municipal, not voluntary, institutions. And so, the AHA turned to the immediate challenge of formulating a model for voluntary hospital planning that the association could juxtapose to liberal reformers' proposals for federally regulated hospital expansion.

The Commission on Hospital Care. With the assistance of the Kellogg Foundation, the Commonwealth Fund, and the National Foundation for Infantile Paralysis, the AHA assembled a planning commission in 1944, the Commission on Hospital Care, to formulate a blueprint for the postwar expansion of the U.S. hospital industry (Stevens 1989, 211). The AHA had one overriding interest in hospital planning. This was to remove the issue of federally sponsored hospital construction from the controversy surrounding national health insurance. Liberal Democrats routinely called attention to widespread and enduring gaps in the geographical distribution of civilian hospitals and cited them as evidence for the need of a comprehensive health program. Ostensibly, national health insurance was the logical cornerstone of such a federal initiative. But the uneven distribution of hospitals was a live concern for legislators of all political stripes. The AHA was determined to enlist the backing of Republicans and southern Democrats for separate measures authorizing federal subsidies for hospital construction—municipal and voluntary—to lessen the rationale for more sweeping interventions into hospital financing and organization.

The AHA sought to preempt any movement toward direct federal regulation of hospital care. In this endeavor, the allegiance of the United States Public Health Service proved to be of capital importance. The USPHS carried most of burden of the Commission on Hospital Care's research efforts and dedicated field personnel to organize or assist the implementation of hospital surveys in over twenty states. The USPHS-sponsored hospital surveys implied that state governments could be set in motion by federal grants-in-aid and could knowingly establish priorities for new construction. The commission's orchestration of cooperative planning efforts among the AHA, the USPHS, and state governments had immediate effect. It proved instrumental in piloting the AHA-sponsored Hospital Survey and Construction Act (Hill-Burton) through Congress in 1945 and 1946. And, the USPHS's approval of Hill-Burton afforded the legislation the pivotal endorsement of the federal agency charged with supervising the program.

The commission's findings and recommendations, entitled *Hospital Care in the United States,* appeared in 1947, a year after the enactment of Hill-Burton (Commission on Hospital Care 1947). *Hospital Care in the United States* represented an odd amalgam of two opposing visions of the U.S. hospital system. One of them was the inspiration of the surgeon general of the USPHS, Thomas Parran. The other represented the thinking of the AHA. Both perspectives were made transparent in congressional deliberations over Hill-Burton. In the first instance, Thomas Parran presented a detailed plan for integrating and coordinating the nation's health services. The Parran model argued for globalizing the role of general hospitals in the delivery of health services and, by implication, for doing away with the institutional boundaries separating the treatment of acute illnesses—the principal domain of municipal and voluntary hospitals—from other health problems for which state governments had normally assumed responsibility: nervous and mental illnesses; tuberculosis; contagious diseases; afflictions requiring chronic or convalescent care; and physical disabilities remedied by long-term rehabilitation. Parran's call for merging curative, preventive, and palliative health care into single sites—local general hospitals—would have brought voluntary hospitals into immediate contact with diseases and patients that had historically remained outside the orbit of the private hospital economy.

The surgeon general's proposed horizontal integration of health services was the first of two major recommendations for achieving economies of scale and scope in hospital care. The second introduced the notion of vertical coordination, beginning from the ranking of hospitals by technological sophistication and capacity for specialized treatment: tertiary hospitals devoted to teaching and research; secondary, or regional, hospitals affording a nearly comprehensive array of conventional specialty care; and primary care hospitals. Each class of hospital would benefit a progressively larger constituency with the smaller, primary care hospitals servicing local populations and the most advanced research hospitals providing leading edge treatments for an entire state. Such a ranking would ostensibly dampen the tendency for local hospitals to needlessly duplicate specialty care services. State regulation was integral to Parran's conception of a rationally planned hospital system. A singular coordinating authority would need to determine the kind of services that individual hospitals would be permitted to develop. In many respects, Canada's public hospital system approximated the Parran model. This was made possible by provincially mandated universal admissions to all general hospitals receiving compulsory provincial-municipal subsidies. And, in many provinces, these policies were teamed with explicit directives requiring general hospitals to give care to those who, in the United States, were otherwise routed to government-owned special disease hospitals. But state governments did not generally possess the fiscal and regulatory leverage over municipal and voluntary hospitals that was so pronounced in the Canadian provinces.

The states had not made any efforts to bridge the divisions within the hospital industry that became entrenched in the nineteenth and early twentieth centuries. For the present, local governments and voluntary institutions held onto control over their separate dominions within the hospital establishment. Parran was at a loss to identify any historical processes at work that were moving local hospital enterprising in the direction of his proposed reorganization. Even the most recent federal and state policies had reaffirmed the distinctive vocations of public and private hospitals. Large-scale investments in government hospitals witnessed during the depression—mostly confined to state-owned mental hospitals, tuberculosis sanatoria, and municipal hospitals for the poor—reasserted the conventional division of labor in the hospital field. New Deal public assistance programs gave state governments no incentives to assume responsibility for the hospital needs of the poor, and they indefinitely postponed the arrival of cooperative ventures between state and local governments and voluntary hospitals. As for employment-based insurance, the hospital-controlled Blue Cross plans had no plausible role in coordinating and integrating health services, excluding as they did primary care, preventative health services, and long-term care. Historical trends did not foreshadow any convergence with the Parran model without radical federal intervention into hospital financing and concurrent mandates to wrest from the states bona fide leadership in hospital planning. The surgeon general wrongly anticipated that comparatively modest federal sanctions would eventually translate into positive state governance of postwar investments in hospital expansion.

In contrast to the surgeon general's revolutionary prospectus for an integrated and coordinated hospital system, the AHA articulated a vision of the postwar hospital order that preserved to the greatest extent the foundations of the prewar hospital establishment—local sovereignty over hospital endeavors with municipal and voluntary institutions operating in symbiotic fashion. It was difficult to read into the AHA's endorsements of conserving the two-tiered hospital systems of the United States's cities—municipal hospitals for the poor and voluntary hospitals for the self-supporting—a surpassing interest in merging the functions of public and private institutions so that a unitary hospital system might result. The AHA recommended that federal and state governments facilitate and supplement, but not supplant, local initiative. In the localities, municipal governments would remain faithful to their historical obligation to provide for the hospital needs of the poor. Private patients would remain the separate lifeblood of voluntary hospitals, now secured through the various branches of employment-based insurance. Coordination between municipal and voluntary institutions would be locally engineered and noncompulsory. Voluntary hospitals would remain dedicated to the advancement of highly specialized medical care and to making it readily available in every community. The surgeon general's proposed vertical hierarchies in the hospital industry plainly did no service to the AHA's conception of locally self-governed hospital regimes.

The area of agreement between the surgeon general and the AHA concerned the approaching expansion of hospital construction beyond the city landscape. In rural, semirural, and suburban locales, economies of scale would not the permit the classical segregation of hospitals projects into freestanding municipal and voluntary institutions. Both the USPHS and the AHA rightly anticipated that this new generation of local hospitals—municipal and voluntary—would have to combine the functions previously divided between them. Thus cooperative arrangements between voluntary and municipal agencies were a practical necessity. Voluntary hospitals would increasingly have to resort to public subsidies to offset the costs of treating public dependents in the absence of nearby special-purpose municipal hospitals for the poor. Municipal hospitals would increasingly rely on income from private patients and would have to develop working relationships with nonprofit and commercial insurance carriers. It was this realization that would prove to be one of the catalysts for transforming the political aspirations of the AHA, presaging the creation of Medicare and Medicaid in the 1960s. The AHA's initially tepid calls for institutionalizing public subsidies to voluntary hospitals for the care of the poor—first articulated on the eve of World War II—took on a newfound sense of urgency in the midst of postwar hospital expansion.

The final report of the Commission on Hospital Care paid homage to the surgeon general's conception of optimal hospital care and to his essential recommendations on such matters as the regional planning of hospital services and the integration of preventative and curative services within general hospitals. However, the commission dismissed Parran's request for instituting mandatory state planning and returned to the familiar AHA precept of stateless coordination of hospital endeavors. Hospital planning, argued the final report, could be accomplished by voluntary bodies comprised of representatives of the hospital professions, organized medicine, and interested members of the public at large. No mention was made of state and local government authority to coordinate voluntary hospital services. Even these diluted testimonials to hospital planning arrived as a dead letter. The AHA had already come away from Hill-Burton with everything it wanted: public subsidies for hospital construction without any manifest threat of federal or state regulation; a benign federal commitment to state licensing laws; and consideration of public investments in the expanding hospital industry withdrawn from deliberations over national health insurance. Hill-Burton had vitiated the political motives for voluntary hospitals to observe any pretense of hospital planning.

Hill-Burton. The Hill-Burton Act followed in the footsteps of the Lanham Act. Hill-Burton made federal matching grants available for constructing both public and voluntary hospitals, and the program subsequently subsidized the construction of more nonprofit hospitals than municipal hospitals. Like Lanham, Hill-Burton made no allowance for federal supervision of assisted hospitals. Congress set aside Surgeon General Parran's recommendations for publicly coordinated hospital expansion; the legislation divorced publicly financed construction from any systemic notions of hospital planning. Hill-Burton made no provision for establishing state regulations to coordinate hospital care with other health services as a condition for receiving federal aid. The law only required state governments to conduct surveys, to establish building priorities, and to clear applicants for federal assistance. Congress did not oblige state legislatures to supervise hospital construction not funded under the act. Hospital planning was left to the discretion of voluntary hospitals and to the volition of state and local governments. Hill-Burton aimed to establish hospitals—public or nonprofit—in the underserved regions of the country, nothing more. And, state governments did not make any concerted efforts to institute any forms of hospital planning independently of the narrow requirements of Hill-Burton (U.S. Department of Health, Education, and Welfare 1960).

Even though Congress did not compel state governments to license hospitals other than those receiving federal assistance, the enactment of Hill-Burton still afforded the AHA the opportunity to push forward with its licensing initiative. Hill-Burton called for a bare minimum of state regulation to promote hospital construction, but these powers greatly exceeded the preexisting regulatory base in the vast majority of states. As of 1937, an AHA study of hospital law found that only three states had recently joined ranks with New York in requiring state approval for the incorporation of new hospitals (American Hospital Association 1937). As of 1945, only Colorado and Rhode Island had licensing laws prescribing minimum standards for all general hospitals. To become eligible for federal grants, state legislatures convened to approve enabling legislation to initiate hospital surveys and to establish administrative responsibility for allocating federal subsidies. It was these legislative sessions that provided the vehicle for realizing the AHA's licensing agenda. The AHA prepared a model licensing act for state legislators in conjunction with the passage of Hill-Burton. The association successfully lobbied the Council of State Governments to endorse the AHA model bill as a means for fulfilling the licensing requirements of Hill-Burton and for instituting state licensing of all acute-care hospitals (American Hospital Association 1947). The AHA had accomplished a long-frustrated ambition in one fell swoop by riding the coattails of federal grants-in-aid legislation.

The AHA model law uniformly adopted by state legislatures avoided any provisions that might be confused with state-mandated hospital planning. The AHA law clearly limited state authority to enforcing minimum standards of operation. The licensing advisory boards provided for in the legislation—consisting of hospital administrators, representatives of the medical profession, and other health professions—would bear the responsibility of developing hospital standards in reference to the prevailing norms of the American Medical Association, the American College of Surgeons, and other voluntary accrediting bodies. There was no express or implied reference to any independent state authority to prescribe regulations concerning the financing, management, or services of voluntary hospitals. The AHA law had no greater ambition than to create a legal basis for closing substandard institutions—mostly for-profit hospitals competing with voluntary hospitals for private patients.

Hill-Burton was an important milestone in U.S. hospital policy. First, it represented the first large-scale attempt to institutionalize government subsidies to voluntary hospitals in the twentieth century. Ever since the late nineteenth century—when state constitutions first outlawed subsidies to private hospitals and progressive urban reformers began their extensive campaign to abolish municipal funding of voluntary hospitals—state and local governments had overwhelmingly earmarked tax funds for hospital purposes to institutions under public ownership and control. Until World War II, federal legislators had followed the same precedent. In arranging hospital care for veterans of military service—one of the few groups for which the federal government acknowledged direct responsibility—Congress had consistently opted to construct and maintain hospitals under federal ownership. Public works projects launched during the New Deal had recapitalized government-owned hospitals as voluntary hospitals struggled to remain solvent. In the 1930s and early 1940s, the national hospital associations dreaded federal intervention in hospital financing because it had historically benefited public hospitals. However, the hospital lobbies discovered that those who steered congressional committees had no desire to create a nationalized hospital system. Congressional leadership was not intent on remaking hospital care for the civilian population but simply on enlarging it in unreconstructed form. Voluntary hospitals would continue to operate as independent enterprises, immune from public regulation. Hill-Burton did not represent a challenge to the institutional motif of the U.S. hospital industry: privately financed, unsupervised hospital care for the self-supporting and publicly financed hospital care for the poor. In this respect, Hill-Burton presaged all national hospital reforms to follow in the postwar era.

Second, Hill-Burton represented a significant turning point in the strategic political behavior of the AHA. Before World War II, the AHA had been an ardent defender of local sovereignty over publicly financed hospital care. From this point forward, the association would endeavor to mold state and local policy through the medium of federal legislation. The AHA had exhorted its state affiliates to lobby for hospital licensing since the 1930s with little prospect of success. It was the passage of Hill-Burton that afforded the AHA the opportunity to have its licensing drive acknowledged and acted upon in state legislatures, circumventing the state associations in toto. For the AHA, the problem was not just that of prolonged municipal sovereignty over hospital policy and of state legislators' habitual disinterest in the finances and management of acute-care hospitals. It was state hospital associations normally exerting little influence over state legislators or over their own membership. Since the AHA generally opposed public regulation of hospital enterprising and defended the institutional prerogatives of voluntary hospitals as preeminently private organizations, it also had to contend with the glaring absence of collective mobilization among voluntary hospitals to sway state and local policy making. The apparent lesson of Hill-Burton for the AHA was that the association had done well to press federal legislators to orchestrate state hospital policy. Henceforth, the AHA would seek to work through Congress to have its legislative ambitions imprinted on state and local governments.

Federal Funding, State Administration, Private Insurance, and the Poor

As President Truman's plan for national health insurance headed for a lopsided defeat, the AHA endeavored to gain congressional support for legislation that would augment tax-supported hospital care for those excluded from employment-based coverage, enlarge the operations of Blue Cross, and accelerate and simplify state and local subsidies to voluntary hospitals. As with the Lanham Act and the attendant passage of Hill-Burton, the EMIC program awakened the AHA to new possibilities for federal spending on hospital care. The Emergency Maternity and Infant Care program was another example of federal subsidies for civilian hospitals without federal regulation. State officials administered the payments for the federal government, and EMIC reimbursed municipal and voluntary hospitals according to their average daily costs. A federally funded, state-administered program modeled after EMIC, but applied to the problem of uncompensated care, captivated the imagination of the national hospital associations. It held out the prospect of breaking down the complex institutional barriers to government subsidies for private hospitals at state and local levels. Federal legislators had proven that they could generate state capacity for channeling public subsidies for private hospital construction with Hill-Burton. Federal legislators might prove themselves equally capable of mobilizing state legislatures to subsidize voluntary hospitals for the care of the poor.

AHA demands for liberalizing subsidies to voluntary hospitals had been roundly ignored for over a decade. The inertia of government spending on municipal hospitals, combined with voluntary hospitals' historical determination to ensure that public hospitals confined their services to the needs of the poor, had imposed formidable constraints on any rapid escalation of state and local subsidies for private hospitals. Federal grants-in-aid of public assistance, if anything, vitiated incentives to incorporate hospital subsidies into state and local welfare programs launched during the New Deal. Even where states and localities had made legal provision for purchasing hospital care for welfare recipients, low payments and bureaucratic headaches deterred voluntary hospitals from seeking compensation from welfare officials. The administrative protocols governing reimbursement were generally so expensive and time consuming that hospitals commonly avoided public payment schemes rather than suffer protracted negotiations over eligibility requirements and allowable costs. Typically, responsibilities for affording hospital care to the poor divided into as many as a dozen agencies with differing eligibility requirements and diverse payment mechanisms. Some public hospitalization plans provided for service in public hospitals only; others allowed for payments to private hospitals; and others still made unrestricted cash payments to welfare recipients who then had an individual responsibility to pay for hospital care out of their own pockets. Various combinations of all three methods within individual state agencies were routinely observed (Sturges 1944; White 1952a; American Hospital Association 1945–46). State governments had created an abundance of administrative channels for financing the hospital needs of the poor. From the perspective of hospital administrators, it was an overabundance that proved self-defeating.

Hill-Aiken. The American Hospital Association coauthored an insurance reform bill with Democratic senator Lister Hill and Republican senator George Aiken (U.S. Senate Subcommittee of the Committee on Labor and Public Welfare 1949, 438–69; U.S. Department of Health, Education, and Welfare 1958, 10–11). Introduced in 1949, the Hill-Aiken Bill endeavored to authorize federal grants to the states to pay the hospital costs of those excluded from private insurance. The working poor would be eligible for assistance as well as beneficiaries of income-maintenance programs. In each state, low-income workers would submit to a means test and pay a percentage of their wages into a state fund. These income taxes would then be pooled with federal, state, and local contributions on behalf of recipients of public assistance into a consolidated insurance fund. The state agency responsible for administering the insurance fund would then authorize regional Blue Cross plans to issue memberships cards to designated beneficiaries. Blue Cross would not assume any financial risk for hospital costs under Hill-Aiken but rather would act as an administrative and a fiscal intermediary. Blue Cross plans would process hospital reimbursement claims, pay the hospitals on behalf of the state, and levy additional charges against the state fund to offset any incidental administrative expenses. Hospitals would bill their average costs per patient day, and the state fund would make good the amount.

Hill-Aiken promised to shore up the market share of Blue Cross, to give substance to the nonprofit carrier's claim of operating for community-wide benefit, and to do away with byzantine claims administration of state and local agencies. Ostensibly, the working poor and public dependents would have obtained publicly financed, privately administered insurance as a gateway to mainstream hospital care. The poor would come to post financial gains rather than losses for voluntary hospitals. The proposed legislation implicitly presented an opportunity to break down the historical division of labor between voluntary and public hospitals without jeopardizing what the AHA perceived to be the commercial foundations of the voluntary hospital sector—private, employment-based hospital insurance. The poor would have gained access to voluntary hospitals. Public hospitals could have extended their services to the working population as voluntary hospitals extended their services to the poor. If enacted, Hill-Aiken would have alleviated the widespread confusion surrounding publicly supported hospital care. All local hospitals—public or private—would have freed themselves from the labor of identifying which government agencies were responsible for underwriting hospital care for the varied classes of public dependents. For the working poor, Hill-Aiken would have relieved hospital administrators of the burdens of investigating the personal finances of those seeking charitable assistance and of collecting nominal payments from them.

In the 1940s and early 1950s, legislative measures like Hill-Aiken failed to attract the requisite political backing for enactment. Even though President Truman withheld his endorsement from anything less than national health insurance, it was Congress that postponed the arrival of tax-supported insurance for those excluded from employment-based hospital plans. Congressional Republicans and southern Democrats possessed the votes to defeat national health insurance. Consistent with their general legislative efforts to stem federal regulatory powers accumulated from the New Deal and the mobilization, Republicans and southern Democrats were not willing to expand federal authority so as to bestow privately administered insurance on the poor. And so, the immediate price of the AHA's alliance with congressional opponents of national health insurance was to set back the hospital lobbies' efforts to win government subsidies for voluntary insurance. As for liberal Democrats, the national hospital associations had alienated them from their cause. Liberal Democrats had endeavored to assure the hospital lobbies that national health insurance would neither jeopardize the institutional prerogatives of voluntary hospitals nor challenge their dominant position within the hospital industry. But the national hospital associations interpreted universal health insurance as the deathblow to voluntarism, and they dramatized national health insurance as socialism. These cold war polemics postponed an entente between the hospital lobbies and liberal congressional reformers. Indignant from such broadsides, liberal Democrats refused to support the American Hospital Association's coveted Hill-Aiken Bill and all other legislative attempts to institutionalize federal subsidies for private insurance in the 1940s and 1950s.

Undeterred, the AHA would not surrender its political efforts to win congressional approval for federal spending to renew publicly sponsored hospital care for the poor. Hospital finance in the United States had always been an ongoing combination of private and public funding. The AHA was content that its opposition to national health insurance succeeded and that employment-based insurance would provide a modern foundation for the private hospital economy. But the association was no less determined to speed the reconstruction of the public hospital economy, providing that voluntary hospitals and the Blue Cross plans became the primary beneficiaries of reform. The riddle for voluntary hospitals became how their customary immunities from public regulation could be made consistent with extending private insurance to all who wanted it but were otherwise disqualified from it. The AHA's proposed solution was that federal, state, and local governments should patronize voluntary insurance like any other private subscriber. To state the matter in these terms, voluntary hospitals and the Blue Cross plans were not prepared to recognize any democratic standards to which they should be held accountable for accepting government subsidies. And so, the hospital lobbies were inclined to blame the inequities of hospital insurance markets on legislators who were unwilling to act as "responsible" purchasers of privately administered insurance on behalf of the poor. Liberal congressional reformers were noticeably unimpressed with this argument.

Notwithstanding their differences, the hospital lobbies and liberal Democrats would eventually make a series of compromises in response to the emerging realities of postwar hospital financing that would make them political allies in the reconstruction of the public hospital economy. In the 1950s, liberal Democrats would reluctantly abandon their campaign for national health insurance with the spread of employment-based insurance to the majority of the working population. They refocused their energies on securing federally sponsored hospital insurance for the beneficiaries of income-maintenance programs. And, they became gradually acclimated to hospital demands for incorporating the Blue Cross plans as fiscal and administrative intermediaries into prospective legislation for establishing a national hospital program. Correspondingly, the AHA and Blue Cross would renounce their faith in state and local governments serving as the primary conduits for channeling public funding to voluntary hospitals for patients excluded from employer-financed coverage. The hospital lobbies would also concede the apparent necessity of institutionalizing compulsory hospital insurance for old-age pensioners through payroll taxes. The AHA's and Blue Cross's approaching endorsements of federal sovereignty over publicly sponsored hospital care also derived from the anticipated consequences of federal grants-in-aid of hospital construction. The AHA's championship of the Hill-Burton program—combined with the advancing integration of municipal hospitals into the economy of private insurance—triggered a commercial transformation of the public hospital sector. This dramatically broadened voluntary hospitals' liabilities for the care of those stranded from employment-based insurance. In the absence of adequate subsidies from state and local governments, the hospital lobbies became inevitably drawn into an alliance with liberal Democrats to engineer a more commanding solution to the problem of the uninsured. The AHA and Blue Cross would defect from the conservative political coalition opposed to federal authority over publicly sponsored hospital care.

The Rise of Federal Sovereignty over Hospital Policy

By the late 1950s and early 1960s, the American Hospital Association and Blue Cross began to reconsider their position on hospital reform. During the 1940s, they had sought national funding for state and local initiatives to address the hospital needs of the poor. The AHA and Blue Cross progressively abandoned their opposition to direct federal jurisdiction over publicly financed hospital benefits. The ongoing public debate over government-financed hospital care largely revolved around the unenviable fate of pensioners. But it was not just the inadequacy of insurance coverage for the elderly that propelled the AHA and Blue Cross to endorse federal sovereignty over hospital policy. Three trends in the postwar hospital economy handed to Congress the lead role in reconstructing hospital programs for public dependents: established patterns of competition within hospital insurance markets, the relative decline of state and local spending on hospital care, and the commercial transformation of municipal hospitals.

The Limits of Private Insurance. The financial limits of private hospital insurance and associated concerns about the diminishing stature of Blue Cross led the AHA to reevaluate federally mandated social insurance for the hospital care of pensioners. The AHA had previously opposed any form of compulsory hospital insurance, fearing it would provide the entering wedge for the creation of universal hospital insurance. This reversal coincided with the perception that private insurance was exhausting its potential for underwriting hospital expenses. Between 1948 and 1962, the percentage of hospital costs met by voluntary insurance rose from 27 percent to 69 percent and then in 1963 fell for the first time to 67 percent (Reed 1964). By 1965, private insurance payments had dropped another 4 points to 63 percent of total hospital income (table 5.2). And, the future of Blue Cross seemed uncertain. Community rating had progressively handicapped Blue Cross in competition with commercial carriers using experience rating. Initially, Blue Cross offered the same premiums to all subscribers. As for-profit carriers entered the hospital insurance market, they offered lower premiums to groups of younger, healthier workers enrolled in employer-sponsored health plans. Consequently, Blue Cross found itself confronted with the problem of adverse selection as its risk pool was increasingly dominated by groups requiring more, not less, hospitalization. In the early 1950s, Blue Cross premiums subsequently rose faster than commercial insurance rates. Eventually, Blue Cross was forced to resort to experience rating to compete with commercial insurers but envisaged a steady reduction of nonprofit insurance coverage if existing market trends held (Dixon 1959; Starr 1982, 327–31). Government-mandated insurance for the aged, if channeled through Blue Cross plans, promised to reinvigorate the nonprofit carriers and to create new sources of hospital revenue above and beyond the disbursements of private insurance (Stevens 1989, 258–72). In 1962, the AHA and Blue Cross issued a joint statement calling for more federal financing:

> We recommend the earliest possible implementation of a national Blue Cross program for a voluntary non-profit plan available to all persons aged 65 and over. We recognize that governmental assistance is necessary to effectively implement this national proposal . . . through the voluntary prepayment system. Conditional upon the administration of this proposed plan by the voluntary prepayment system, the tax source of funds is of secondary importance to us. (American Hospital Association and Blue Cross Association 1962, 2:28)

Vanishing Public Funding. The second impetus to federal action was the incapacity of state and local governments to afford a minimum standard of hospital care for those of all ages barred from private coverage. In the postwar era, state and local financing of hospital care declined as a percentage of total hospital income. Public funding fell from 24 percent in 1935 to 20 percent in 1950. It slipped to 15 percent in 1958 (table 5.3). Federal programs had done little to stem the erosion of state and local spending on hospital care. In 1950, Congress rewrote the cost-sharing provisions of grants-in-aid of public assistance. These revisions allowed payments to private hospitals for the care of public dependents to qualify for matching funds. But the maximum limits placed on federal contributions to state programs remained so low—$50 per case per month—that state legislators had no incentive to prioritize spending for health care. In most states, county administration was still paramount. The added burdens of meeting federal eligibility requirements—pooling health care assistance appropriations into consolidated health funds—normally canceled out any gains from federal cost sharing (Norman 1952; Greenfield 1957; Commission on Financing Hospital Care 1955, 3:63–77).

The relative decline of public spending on hospital care need not have created undue financial burdens for private hospitals as long as municipal hospitals absorbed most uncompensated care at a greatly reduced cost. However, this was not the case in the 1950s. Federal grants-in-aid of hospital construction recapitalized voluntary hospitals to a greater extent than government-owned hospitals. Between 1940 and 1960, the proportion of acute-care beds in nonfederal public hospitals fell to 25 percent from 30

TABLE 5.2.   Enrollment in Private Hospital Insurance, and Benefit Expenditures as a Percentage of Hospital Income, United States, 1950–65

	1950	1955	1960	1965
Enrollment (in thousands)	79,045	112,755	140,117	164,369
Coverage (as a percentage of population)[a]	51	64	72	79
Benefit expenditures (in millions)	680	1,679	3,304	5,790
As a percentage of hospital income	32	49	59	63

Source: Reed 1967, 12, 22; U.S. Bureau of the Census 1975, B413–22, X957–62.
Note: Nonfederal, short-term general, and allied specialty hospitals.
[a]Figures for enrollment and percentage coverage supplied to U.S. government from the Health Insurance Association of America tended to overestimate enrollment by 3 to 4%.

TABLE 5.3.   Hospital Income by Source, United States, 1935, 1950, and 1958, by Percentage

Source of Income	1935	1950	1958
Taxes	24.4	19.8	15.0
Pay patients[a]	61.9	74.1	80.8
Endowments and gifts	13.7	6.1	4.2

Source: Data from Klarman 1963, 492.
Note: Nonfederal, general, and allied specialty hospitals.
[a]Pay-patient income includes private insurance payments.

percent. Even if municipal hospitals remained loyal to their historical mandate to treat the poor, voluntary hospitals were still facing a relative increase in demands for free and low-cost care. However, the Hill-Burton program for hospital construction inspired a commercial transformation of the public sector. Local-government hospitals constructed under Hill-Burton typically served the entire population of their surrounding communities, not just the poor. The new public hospitals were small, rural, and primarily located in the South, in the West, and in the North-Central states (American Hospital Association 1976). By 1961, public hospitals obtained more than one-half of their aggregate income from paying patients, a stunning departure from prewar times (Hollingsworth and Hollingsworth 1987, 98). The relative decline and commercialization of municipal hospitals added urgency to expanding public subsidies to voluntary hospitals to care for the uninsured (table 5.4).

At the outset of the 1960s, federal attempts to trigger more state and local spending on hospital care were not encouraging. Kerr-Mills legislation further liberalized federal grants-in-aid of health care for the aged but did not dissipate the reluctance of state governments to offset the hospital

TABLE 5.4.   Hospital Income and Capacity, by Ownership, United States, 1958

	Public	Voluntary	Profit	Total
Income (in millions)	1,003	3,538	241	4,782
Source of Income				
Taxes	502	208	5	715
Pay patients[a]	501	3,130	236	3,867
Endowments and gifts	—	200	—	200
	%	%	%	%
Taxes	50.0	5.9	2.1	15.0
Pay patients	50.0	88.4	97.9	80.8
Endowments and gifts	—	5.7	—	4.2
Capacity				
	%	%	%	%
Hospitals	22	60	18	100
Beds	25	69	6	100
Admissions	20	73	7	100

Source: Klarman 1963, 510; American Hospital Association 1959.
Note: Nonfederal, general, and allied specialty hospitals.
[a]Pay-patient income includes private insurance payments.

expenses of the elderly. In the first years of Kerr-Mills funding, the percentage of the aged eligible for health care assistance under state programs actually dropped. This experience discredited the notion that state initiatives would avert the need for unilateral federal action (Stevens and Stevens 1974, 19–41). Private health insurance had matured into a politically unassailable fortress. Closing gaps in hospital insurance coverage would not appear in the guise of a universal program. As far as voluntary hospitals were concerned, employment-based health plans had well served their primary purpose—maximizing the scope of private arrangements for the self-supporting and confining government-sponsored hospital care to the needy. Whatever the shortcomings of this arrangement, the benefit expenditures of market-based insurance had nevertheless been pivotal to the emergence of a well-endowed hospital industry. Before the enactment of Medicare and Medicaid, hospital expenditures per capita in the United States were second only to those of Canada (table 5.5).

Medicare and Medicaid. As a last resort, the federal government enacted Medicare and Medicaid programs in 1965. Without guidance from state or local governments for reconstructing publicly sponsored hospital care, Congress looked to the Social Security Act to provide a model for tax-supported health insurance. Part A of Medicare—compulsory

TABLE 5.5.   Hospital Capacity and Income in Canada and the United States, 1965

	Canada	United States
Hospitals	1,009	4,879
Hospital beds	116,981	694,000
Beds per thousand	6.0	3.6
Admissions	2,988,795	24,618,000
Admissions per thousand	152	127
Patient days	34,925,891	194,180,000
Patients days per thousand	1,778	1,000
Average stay (days)	11.6	7.9
Full-time employees per hundred beds	194	191
Total expenditures (in millions of U.S. dollars)[a]	1,196	8,637
Per capita	61	44
Per patient day	34	44

Source: Statistics Canada 1983, B93–460; U.S. Bureau of the Census 1975, 1:B221–49.
Note: Nonfederal, general, and allied specialty hospitals, governmental and nonprofit.
[a]Canadian dollar figures converted at 1965 exchange rate: 1.00 CAN = $1.08 US.

hospital insurance for pensioners—circumvented state financing and administration. Medicaid primarily expanded federal funding and regulation of state health plans for other beneficiaries of income-maintenance programs, namely, means-tested recipients of public assistance. The secret of these programs' legislative success, as Herman Somers put it, was that "no existing institutions were overturned or seriously threatened by the new law" (Somers 1968, 121). In restricting compulsory hospital insurance to the elderly, Medicare posed no threat to the market in employment-based hospital insurance. Medicare exonerated private underwriters of the hazards of insuring the largest low-income, high-risk group of the population. The program allowed private carriers to serve as intermediaries between federal administrators and local hospitals. Private insurers would assume responsibility for claims processing and reimbursements. Hospitals obtained the privilege of designating the carrier of their choice. And so, Medicare expanded, rather than contracted, the operations of Blue Cross. By allowing hospitals to cost their services unilaterally and to retain private control over hospital accreditation, federal legislators brought hospitals within the orbit of a major public program without any manifest threat of public regulation (Feder 1977).

While Medicare released health care for the aged from the grip of state and local governments, the inclusion of Medicaid in the 1965 Social Security Act amendments had mutually reinforcing logics, ideological and fiscal. The architecture of the Social Security Act provided no unified vehicle for bestowing entitlements. The act recognized the distinction between earned and unearned public benefits. Earned benefits represented a form of social insurance. Recipients claimed assistance as a matter of right without respect to individual circumstances. Benefits as of right were inseparable from earmarked contributions from payroll taxes levied against employers and employees. Public assistance was an unearned benefit, financed from general tax revenue and dependent upon the demonstration of abject need according to means tests. Social insurance fell under the rubric of exclusive federal control or, alternatively, under joint federal-state administration with federal legislators supplying clear-cut fiscal and programmatic leadership. But public assistance descended from the poor laws and gave state legislators more discretion in setting benefit levels and eligibility requirements. The underlying philosophy of the Social Security Act did not betray any predisposition for extending first-rate hospital care to all beneficiaries of income-maintenance programs. And, the fiscally reckless terms of Medicare precluded broadening its base to include other low-income groups (Marmor 1969, 60–61).

Conclusion

The second transformation of the U.S. hospital economy—the decades-long movement to construct a new set of institutions to stabilize hospital budgets through the medium of insurance—reaffirmed the tenets of the pre-depression hospital order: publicly financed arrangements for the poor and privately financed arrangements for the self-supporting. The reconstruction of the private hospital economy gathered momentum from the associated efforts of voluntary hospitals to reassert their dominance over the pay-patient trade and, by correspondence, to reverse the mounting influence of the public hospital system during the 1930s. The hospital-sponsored Blue Cross plans strategically modified the original framework of employment-based health insurance, as articulated in U.S. workers' compensation laws, which alleviated the conflicts of interest between business corporations, insurance companies, the hospital industry, and the medical profession in the making of a reformed health insurance market. Blue Cross laid the groundwork for a commercial alliance between corporate sponsors and health care providers that became the enduring foundation for the political opposition to national health insurance.

The reconstruction of the public hospital economy paralleled the reconstruction of U.S. poor relief. Municipal governments assembled the infrastructure for publicly sponsored hospital care in prewar times, but the local fisc demonstrated little promise for addressing the hospital needs of public dependents after World War II. Lethargic state governments neglected to fill the void created by declining municipal activism, and so the initiative passed to Washington. Congress first attempted, without success, to encourage state governments to assume primary responsibility for the health care of those excluded from employment-based insurance. In the mid-1960s, a last ditch attempt to restore government's historical obligations succeeded with the creation of two federal programs— Medicare for old-age pensioners and Medicaid for recipients of means-tested public assistance. Whereas Canadian legislators found no virtue in linking tax-supported hospital insurance to income-maintenance programs, federal legislators in the United States proved that such a relationship could be forced. It was wrung out of the Social Security Act. The ready-made architecture of the Social Security Act afforded Congress with a fiscal, ideological, and administrative framework for publicly financed hospital insurance and offered an authoritative resolution to the dilemma of federal sovereignty over health policy.

CHAPTER 6

Conclusion

I have argued that the rationalization of hospital policy in the United States and Canada manifested divergent assumptions about public and private responsibilities for arranging hospital care and about the relationship between them. These paradigms imposed different ideological biases on national reforms devoted to standardizing publicly financed hospital insurance in the postwar era. The U.S. paradigm afforded Congress with legitimate grounds for implementing government-sponsored hospital plans for beneficiaries of income-maintenance programs, while the Canadian paradigm motivated the nationwide adoption of universal hospital plans under joint federal-provincial auspices. In each country, these paradigms were, in part, the unanticipated consequences of the social, economic, and political forces that steered the development of nineteenth-century poor relief. In the United States, the prevailing tendency was to divide the financing and management of organized charities into two distinctive branches—one secular and public and the other confessional and private. In Canada, legislators fused them. What consummated these paradigms was the commercial transformation of hospital finance that differentiated acute-care institutions for the sick from the other regiments of the charitable establishment at the turn of the century. As fees became the principal source of income for confessionally based hospitals, U.S. conventions of poor relief abetted the creation of two separate hospital systems—one public and charitable and the other private and commercial. The Canadian preference for uniting the disparate vocations of secular and confessional charity founded a universal hospital system, at once charitable and commercial but accessible to patients of all social classes.

In Canada, the British conquest of New France led to a constitutional settlement that exempted local governments from any formal obligations in the realm of poor relief. The imperial government vested the provincial authorities with undivided responsibility for appropriating public funds for charitable endeavors, and the provinces allocated these expenditures to private charities under confessional management. Since the Crown acknowledged two established churches in the Canadian territories—one

156

Anglican and the other Catholic— local administration of poor relief fell under ecclesiastical control. The advent of home rule made representation from both English Protestants and French Catholics essential to forming stable governments under party rule. Hence, political patronage of confessional charities became more entrenched in legislative practice as the provinces redoubled their efforts to meet pressing needs for charitable assistance stemming from midcentury immigration. Reforming local governments were not deliberately implicated in relief operations during the transition to democratic self-government, but provincial legislators established conventions of municipal rule that would later afford them a vehicle for mobilizing local financing for hospital purposes. In the era of Confederation, the rationalization of hospital policy took for granted the antecedent foundations of Canadian hospital charity: provincial sovereignty over government-financed hospital care and confessional sponsorship of locally organized hospital projects. The routinization of provincial grants to voluntary institutions anticipated legislation standardizing municipal contributions to government-recognized hospitals. These political reforms coincided with, and advanced, the therapeutic and commercial transformation of hospital services. As the benefits of hospital treatment became more universal, mandatory subsidies to local hospitals on behalf of those who could not afford the expense of their care took on newfound significance. Government financing was progressively viewed as the means to insure universal access to the reformed hospitals. In every Canadian jurisdiction, a public hospital system materialized under provincial supervision.

In the United States, colonial instruments of rule delegated control over public charity to local governments. The evangelical bent of American Protestantism retarded investments in confessional charities dedicated to poor relief, and so municipal poorhouses served as the primary locus of institutional care for the sick poor in the antebellum era. The democratization of the American polity carried with it constitutional reforms that inadvertently deprived state legislatures of their authority to finance and supervise the work of voluntary benevolent associations. These measures formally divided the charitable establishment into two branches—one private and the other public. As state governance of charitable corporations disintegrated, midcentury immigration altered the ethnic and religious composition of the settled populace, igniting confessional rivalries that fueled the proliferation of hospital charities under voluntary management in the postbellum era. Parochial charities subsequently became the dominant force in the emerging hospital industry, without the benefit of routine assistance from state or local governments. The commercial transformation of the private hospital economy coincided with the political transformation of local government. In the late nineteenth and early twentieth centuries, the rationalization of municipal poor relief redivided the finances and management of public and private charities in a bid to restore the institutional motif of antebellum philanthropy and so began the conversion of poorhouse infirmaries into freestanding municipal hospitals. Under the direction of urban reformers, the presiding logic of hospital policy was that of segregation. This ethos prompted the formation of a two-tiered hospital industry consisting of public institutions for the poor and private institutions for the self-supporting.

In both countries, the Great Depression prolonged the influence of timeworn hospital policy. In Canada, the economic crisis magnified the importance of government funding to the public hospital system. In the United States, all levels of government enlarged their stock in publicly owned hospitals during the 1930s, exaggerating the commercial bias of the surviving organizations within the private hospital system. Rather than portend a radical break from the past, the depression gave new currency to established patterns of government-financed hospital care.

The postwar reconstruction of the public hospital economy remained faithful to the principles long embedded in provincial statutes and in the standard operating practices of Canadian hospitals. The consolidation of a nationwide system of universal hospital insurance was also an artifact of emergent protocols for setting federal priorities in the realm of hospital finance. Intergovernmental summits became the venues for articulating provincial understandings of the appropriate objects of national policy, and the subsequent enactment of federal legislation came to rest upon the endorsements of a majority of provinces. There were reciprocal channels of influence running between these levels of government. The prospect of obtaining matching federal contributions for hospital insurance also mediated provincial deliberations over reform. It alleviated concerns about the fiscal burdens of realizing universal coverage for those provinces that would have otherwise considered it prohibitively expensive to underwrite comprehensive hospital plans out of their own resources. Nonetheless, the dialectics of Canadian federalism did not consistently favor a national accord on hospital insurance. As the spectacular failure of the Conference on Postwar Reconstruction demonstrated, hospital reforms could be, and were, defeated when paired with other controversial measures. Ultimately, progress on hospital insurance depended on implementing health reforms in stages. Had provincial and federal legislators remained wedded to the notion of introducing government health plans for hospital and medical care as jointly insured services, opposition from the medical profession might have also frustrated advances for compulsory hospital insurance. The decision to postpone negotiations over publicly financed medical benefits greatly improved the chances of reaching a discrete settlement on a national program for hospital care. This incremental approach to health reform allowed hospital policy to serve as a working model for ensuing efforts to universalize medical insurance.

In the United States, hospital policy would not become the opening wedge for national health insurance. The synergy between federal and state governments did not privilege the formation of national standards for universal coverage. Unlike the Canadian parliament, Congress never faced the dilemma of choosing between patronizing universal plans under state direction or limiting federal subsidies for hospital care to the needs of public dependents. The political currents of the nineteenth and early twentieth centuries had conditioned state legislatures to look upon acute-care hospitals as intrinsically local or private concerns. Of the immense variety of political coalitions ruling state governments, not one of them devised a legislative program for universalizing hospital insurance. Only gradually did local sovereignty over hospital policy dissolve in the midst of postwar hospital expansion, and the corresponding routinization of state funding for hospital purposes emerged after voluntary hospitals had waged and won a national battle for private control over hospital insurance. Thus, the states uniformly confined their interests to arranging hospital care for welfare recipients. The hospital federations were not mistaken when they characterized national health insurance as revolutionary and out of keeping with the historical evolution of the U.S. hospital industry. The incipient division of the hospital establishment into two branches—one public and charitable and the other private and commercial—led voluntary hospitals to identify their mission with obtaining maximum allowances for the development of private insurance. It was their profound conviction that universal health plans under public management would violate the sacred conventions of U.S. hospital finance and badly compromise the perceived virtues of private sponsorship of hospital enterprises. These anxieties carried voluntary hospitals to the forefront of the movement to institutionalize employment-based health insurance as a viable alternative to government sovereignty over hospital budgeting. Notwithstanding their deep-seated contempt for universal health insurance, voluntary hospitals became leading advocates for reconstructing tax-supported hospital care for public dependents. The substantial erosion of municipal provisions for the poor after World War II, combined with the glaring inadequacies of state programs, intensified pressures on federal legislators to restore public obligations for underwriting the hospital expenses of those disqualified from market-based coverage. Congress eventually reached into the Social Security Act to find a model for government-sponsored hospital insurance. Medicare and Medicaid reinstated the historical division of labor between public and private financing of hospital care but departed from precedent by normalizing public subsidies for private hospitals.

To the present, U.S. and Canadian lawmakers have not disturbed the basic tenets of health policy, however much they have added new elements to them. In Canada, the terms and conditions of federal subsidies to the provincial health plans have undergone several revisions in the 1970s, 1980s, and 1990s. Provincial governments are increasingly vesting newly formed regional authorities with far-reaching powers to finance, organize, monitor, and supervise hospital care and allied health services. The movement to reinvent localized management of government-sponsored health benefits has accompanied profound shifts in Canadian thinking about the relative contributions of hospital and medical care to health and well-being. A *wellness* paradigm that has steadily gained acceptance in legislative circles primarily traces the origins of good health to environmental factors, lifestyle choices, and social support networks. The rise of therapeutic skepticism—the retreat from an unqualified faith in biomedical approaches to relieving illness—is yielding a growing emphasis on identifying and modifying the social determinants of health. Regionalization has become the chosen instrument for bringing practical definition to a sweeping reform agenda: encouraging civic participation in setting priorities for health care funding; coordinating and integrating community-based and acute-care services; expanding the reach of public health initiatives, mutual assistance, and educational programs devoted to improving living habits; and assembling an organizational vehicle for increasing knowledge about the appropriateness and effectiveness of differing agents of health promotion. In this attempt to strike a proper balance among preventative and remedial services, universal access to hospital care has endured as a guiding principle of contemporary reform.

Just as Canadian legislators generate new institutions for regulating hospital enterprises that afford universal access, U.S. governments have devised ever more complicated legal frameworks for preserving the division of labor between public and private financing of hospital care. The municipal hospitals of antiquity owed their existence to local policymakers who sought to enlarge public control and scrutiny over hospital care in direct, visible ways. The housing of the poor in segregated institutions, however indefensible on other grounds, had this one advantage. With the postwar attrition of the public hospital system and the subsequent privatization of the public hospital economy, federal and state governments were left vulnerable to unchecked hospital inflation in the private sector. This has prompted successive campaigns to rein in public spending and to establish novel forms of government sovereignty over the private hospital economy. The conventional duality of U.S. hospital policy has recently bred a third dimension. There remain two distinctive bodies of law regulating public and private financing of hospital services, the former prescribing the manner of raising and allocating government funds for the hospital needs of public dependents and the latter governing corporate investments in employment-based health plans. Added to these is an expanding legislative domain more specifically concerned with reorganizing the *provision* of hospital benefits as a vehicle for cost control. National and state policies favoring the development of health maintenance organizations, managed care networks, and other forms of corporate supervision over health care providers have, in theory, intensified competition among health plans. These market-based reforms have not yet realized the economies prospectively attributed to them.

President Clinton's health security plan represented an attempt to weave these disparate legislative strands into a comprehensive program for achieving universal coverage and disciplining health care expenditures. The proposed reconstruction of health insurance markets, coupled with government-mandated subscriptions to competing health plans, would have enshrined public sovereignty over health care funding and private sovereignty over health care provision. In simple terms, the initiative called for business corporations to relinquish immediate control over the financing of health benefits for the working population, yet it would have obliged them to bear the greater expense of capitalizing the reformed health care economy. Ultimately, the business establishment refused to endorse these arrangements. U.S. health policy has now returned to its more familiar moorings: ritualistic agonizing over the fiscal burdens of Medicare and Medicaid programs; piecemeal amendments to tax codes and insurance regulations geared to arresting the deterioration of employment-based coverage; and the steady accumulation of legislative measures aimed at speeding the corporate transformation of the health care industry and at curbing the perceived abuses of health services conglomerates. The more things change, the more they stay the same.

Bibliography

Agnew, G. Harvey. 1935. "Governmental Methods of Providing for the Care of the Indigent Sick in Canada as Compared to the Rendition of This Similar Service in the United States." *Transactions of the American Hospital Association* 37:888–902.

——. 1940. *The Hospital System of Canada.* Toronto: Canadian Medical Association.

——. 1974. *Canadian Hospitals, 1920 to 1970: A Dramatic Half Century.* Toronto: University of Toronto Press.

Alberta. 1922. *Revised Statutes.* Edmonton: King's Printer.

——. 1935. *Statutes.* Edmonton: King's Printer.

——. 1938. *The Case for Alberta.* Part 1, *Alberta's Problems and the Dominion-Provincial Relations, Submission to the Royal-Commission on Dominion-Provincial Relations.* Edmonton: King's Printer.

——. 1951. *Statutes.* Edmonton: King's Printer.

Alberta. Legislative Commission on Medical and Health Services. 1934. *Final Report.* Edmonton: King's Printer.

American Hospital Association. 1937. *Incorporation, Taxation and Licensure of Hospitals in the United States.* Chicago: American Hospital Association.

——. 1945–46. "Hospital Care of the Medically Indigent." In *1945 Hospital Review,* 2:39–46. Chicago: American Hospital Association.

——. 1947. *Hospital Licensing Act.* Chicago: American Hospital Association. Mimeographed.

——. 1959. *Hospitals, Guide Issue.* Chicago: American Hospital Association.

——. 1976. *1974 Statistical Profile of Public General Hospitals.* Chicago: American Hospital Association.

American Hospital Association and American Public Welfare Association. 1938. "Hospital Care for the Needy: Relations between Public Authorities and Hospitals." *Hospitals* 12 (8): 17–24.

American Hospital Association and Blue Cross Association. 1962. *Financing Health Care for the Aged.* Vol. 2. Chicago: American Hospital Association and Blue Cross Association.

American Medical Association. Bureau of Medical Economics. 1933. *Medical Relations under Workmen's Compensation.* Chicago: American Medical Association.

American Medical Association. Council on Medical Education and Hospitals.

1928. "Hospital Service in the United States." *Journal of the American Medical Association* 90 (12): 911–22.

―――. 1935. "Hospital Service in the United States." *Journal of the American Medical Association* 104 (13): 1075–85.

―――. 1941. "Hospital Service in the United States." *Journal of the American Medical Association* 116 (11): 1055–70.

Anderson, James D. 1972. "Non-Partisan Urban Politics in Canadian Cities." In *Emerging Party Politics in Urban Canada,* edited by Jack K. Masson and James D. Anderson, 5–25. Toronto: McClelland and Stewart.

Bailyn, Bernard. 1968. *The Origins of American Politics.* New York: Knopf.

Barbour, Levi L., et al. 1901. "The Division of Work between Public and Private Charities: Subsidies." *Proceedings of the National Conference of Charities and Corrections* 28:118–31.

Bell, Douglas. 1959. "Current Developments in Health Insurance in Canada." In *Yearbook of the Canadian Life Insurance Officers Association,* 31–39. Toronto: Canadian Life Insurance Officers Association.

Berger, Peter L., and Thomas Luckmann. 1966. *The Social Construction of Reality: A Treatise in the Sociology of Knowledge.* New York: Doubleday.

Bourinot, John George. 1887. *Local Government in Canada: An Historical Study.* Johns Hopkins University Studies in History and Political Science, vols. 5 and 6. Baltimore: Johns Hopkins University.

Bremner, Robert H. 1980. *The Public Good: Philanthropy and Welfare in the Civil War Era.* New York: Knopf.

British Columbia. 1911. *Revised Statutes.* Victoria: King's Printer.

―――. 1938. *British Columbia in the Canadian Confederation, Submission to the Royal Commission on Dominion-Provincial Relations.* Victoria: King's Printer.

―――. 1948. *Statutes.* Victoria: King's Printer.

British Columbia. Department of the Provincial Secretary. 1926–36. *Annual Hospital Reports.* Victoria: King's Printer.

British Columbia. Royal Commission on State Health Insurance and Maternity Benefits. 1929–1930. *Transcript of Evidence.* Vol. 2. Victoria: King's Printer.

―――. 1932. *Final Report.* Victoria: King's Printer.

Bryce, James. 1891. *The American Commonwealth.* Vol. 1. New York: Macmillan.

Canada. 1945. *Health, Welfare and Labour: Reference Book for Dominion-Provincial Conference on Reconstruction.* Ottawa: King's Printer.

Canada. Advisory Committee on Health Insurance. 1943. *Report.* Ottawa: King's Printer.

Canada, Bureau of Statistics. 1928. *The Canada Year Book, 1927–28.* Ottawa: King's Printer.

―――. 1936. *The Canada Year Book, 1934–35.* Ottawa: King's Printer.

―――. 1957. *Hospital Statistics.* Vol. 1. Ottawa: Queen's Printer.

―――. 1958. *National Accounts, Income and Expenditure, 1926–56.* Ottawa: Queen's Printer.

Canada. Department of National Health and Welfare. 1958. *Voluntary Hospital and Medical Insurance in Canada, 1956.* Ottawa: Queen's Printer.

———. 1960. *Hospital Care in Canada: Recent Trends and Developments.* Ottawa: Queen's Printer.

Canada. Royal Commission on Dominion-Provincial Relations. 1940a. *Report.* Book 1. Ottawa: King's Printer.

———. 1940b. *Recommendations.* Book 2. Ottawa: King's Printer.

Canada. Statistics Canada. 1983. *Historical Statistics of Canada.* 2d ed. Ottawa: Government Printing Center.

Canadian Hospital Council. 1937. *Transactions.* Toronto: Canadian Hospital Council.

———. 1942. *Principles of Health Insurance as They Relate to Hospitals.* Bulletin of the Canadian Hospital Council, no. 41.

———. 1943. *Hospitals and Health Insurance: A Presentation to the Special Committee on Social Security of the House of Commons.* Bulletin of the Canadian Hospital Council, no. 43.

Careless, J. M. S. 1967. *The Union of the Canadas: The Growth of Canadian Institutions, 1841–1867.* Toronto: McClelland and Stewart.

Carpenter, Niles. 1930. *Hospital Services for Patients of Moderate Means: A Study of Certain American Hospitals.* Committee on the Costs of Medical Care, publication no. 4. Washington, DC: Committee on the Costs of Medical Care.

Casidy, Harry M. 1945. *Public Health and Welfare Reorganization: The Postwar Problem in the Canadian Provinces.* Toronto: Ryerson Press.

Catholic Hospital Council of Canada. 1942. *The Catholic Hospital Council of Canada and Health Insurance: A Brief for Presentation before the Select Committee of the House of Commons and the Senate of Canada.* Mimeographed.

Coler, Bird S. 1899. *Municipal Subsidies to Private Charities, Being a Report to the Board of Estimate and Apportionment.* New York: Martin Brown.

———. 1901. *Municipal Government as Illustrated by the Charter, Finances, and Public Charities of New York.* New York: Appleton.

Commission on Financing Hospital Care. 1955. *Financing Hospital Care for Non-wage and Low-Income Groups.* Vol. 3, *Financing Hospital Care in the United States.* New York: McGraw-Hill.

Commission on Hospital Care. 1947. *Hospital Care in the United States.* New York: Commonwealth Fund.

Committee on the Costs of Medical Care. 1928. *The Five-Year Program of the Committee on the Costs of Medical Care.* Publication no. 1. Washington, DC: Committee on the Costs of Medical Care.

———. 1932. *Medical Care for the American People.* Chicago: University of Chicago Press.

Cox, W. E. 1951. "Financing Indigents and Near Indigents." *Canadian Hospital* 28 (12): 34, 78.

Crawford, Kenneth Grant. 1954. *Canadian Municipal Government.* Toronto: University of Toronto Press.

Davis, Michael M. 1932. "The Committee on the Costs of Medical Care Makes Its Report." *Modern Hospital* 39 (12): 41–46.

Davis, Michael M., and C. Rufus Rorem. 1932. *The Crisis in Hospital Finance.* Chicago: University of Chicago Press.

Dealy, James. 1914. *The Growth of American State Constitutions: From 1776 to the End of the Year 1914.* Boston: Athenian Press.

Denison, Edward F. 1942. "Consumer Expenditures for Selected Groups of Services, 1929–41." *Survey of Current Business* 22 (10): 23–30.

DiMaggio, Paul J., and Walter W. Powell. 1991. "Introduction." In *The New Institutionalism in Organizational Analysis,* edited by Walter W. Powell and Paul J. Dimaggio, 1–38. Chicago: University of Chicago Press.

Dixon, James P. 1959. "The Hospital's Viewpoint." *American Journal of Public Health* 49 (2): 176–80.

Dobbin, Frank. 1994. *Forging Industrial Policy: The United States, Britain, and France in the Railway Age.* New York: Cambridge University Press.

Falk, I. S. 1936. *Security against Sickness: A Study of Health Insurance.* New York: Doubleday.

Falk, I. S., Margaret C. Klem, and Nathan Sinai. 1933. *The Incidence of Illness and the Receipt and Costs of Medical Care among Representative Families: Experience in Twelve Consecutive Months 1928–1931.* Committee on the Costs of Medical Care, publication no. 26. Chicago: University of Chicago Press.

Feder, Judith. 1977. *Medicare: The Politics of Federal Hospital Insurance.* Lexington, MA: Lexington Books.

Frankel, Emil. 1925. *State-Aided Hospitals in Pennsylvania.* Bulletin no. 25. Harrisburg: Pennsylvania Department of Public Charities.

Glaser, William A. 1970. *Social Settings and Medical Organization: A Cross-National Study of the Hospital.* New York: Atherton.

Goldwater, S. S. 1909. "The Appropriation of Public Funds for the Partial Support of Voluntary Hospitals in the United States and Canada." *Transactions of the American Hospital Association* 11:242–94.

———. 1935. "Discussion on Papers Presented." *Transactions of the American Hospital Association* 37:909–10.

———. 1949. *On Hospitals.* New York: Macmillan.

Graham, Roger. 1990. *Old Man Ontario: Leslie Frost.* Toronto: University of Toronto Press.

Grauer, A. E. 1939. *Public Health: A Study Prepared for the Royal Commission on Dominion-Provincial Relations.* Ottawa: King's Printer.

Greenfield, Margaret. 1957. *Medical Care for Welfare Recipients: State Programs.* Berkeley: University of California, Bureau of Public Administration.

Greenhaus, Brereton. 1968. "Paupers and Poor Houses: The Development of Poor Relief in Early New Brunswick." *Social History/Histoire Sociale* 1:103–28.

Griffith, Ernest S. 1974. *A History of American City Government: The Conspicuous Failure, 1870–1900.* New York: Praeger.

Hall, Peter A. 1986. *Governing the Economy.* Cambridge: Polity Press.

———. 1993. "Policy Paradigms, Social Learning and the State." *Comparative Politics* 25 (3): 275–96.

Hamilton, James A. 1943. "The Future of the Voluntary Hospital," *Hospitals* 17 (6): 12–17.

Hart, George. 1958. "Death of the Poor Law in Nova Scotia." *Canadian Welfare* 34 (5): 226–32.

Hitchcock, Henry. 1887. *American State Constitutions: A Study of Their Growth.* New York: Putnam's Sons.

Hodgetts, J. E. 1955. *Pioneer Public Service: An Administrative History of the United Canadas, 1841–1867.* Toronto: University of Toronto Press.

Hollingsworth, J. Rogers, and Ellen Jane Hollingsworth. 1987. *Controversy about American Hospitals: Funding, Ownership, and Performance.* Washington, DC: American Enterprise Institute.

Jamieson, Stuart. 1957. *Industrial Relations in Canada.* Ithaca: Cornell University Press.

Johnson, Arlien. 1931. *Public Policy and Private Charities.* Chicago: University of Chicago Press.

Jones, Arthur W., and Francisca K. Thomas. 1938. *Hospital Survey for New York.* Vol. 3. New York: United Hospital Fund.

Katz, Michael B. 1986. *In the Shadow of the Poorhouse: A Social History of Welfare in America.* New York: Basic Books.

Kingsdale, Jon M. 1981. "The Growth of Hospitals: An Economic History in Baltimore." Ph.D. diss., University of Michigan.

Klarman, Herbert E. 1963. *Hospital Care in New York City: The Roles of Voluntary and Municipal Hospitals.* New York: Columbia University Press.

Kuhn, Thomas. 1970. *The Structure of Scientific Revolutions.* Chicago: University of Chicago Press.

Lapp, John A., and Dorothy Ketcham. 1926. *Hospital Law.* Milwaukee: Bruce Publishing.

Lincoln, Charles Z. 1906. *A Constitutional History of New York.* Vol. 4. Rochester, NY: Lawyers Co-operative Publishing.

Lipset, Seymour Martin. 1990. *Continental Divide: The Values and Institutions of the United States and Canada.* New York: Routledge.

Manitoba. 1913. *Revised Statutes.* Winnipeg: King's Printer.

———. 1933. *Revised Statutes.* Winnipeg: King's Printer.

March, James G., and Johan P. Olsen. 1989. *Rediscovering Institutions: The Organizational Basis of Politics.* New York: Free Press.

Marmor, Theodore. 1969. "The Congress: Medicare Politics and Policy." In *American Political Institutions and Public Policy,* edited by Alan P. Sindler, 3–66. Boston: Little, Brown.

Martin, Paul, Sr. 1985. *A Very Public Life.* Vol. 2. Toronto: Deneau Publishers.

Millon, David. 1990. "Theories of the Corporation." *Duke Law Journal* 193:201–62.

Mountin, Joseph, Elliot H. Pennell, and Evelyn Flook. 1938. *Selected Character-*

istics of Hospital Facilities in 1936. Public Health Bulletin, no. 243, part 1. Washington, DC: USGPO.

Mountin, Joseph, Elliot H. Pennell, and Kay Pearson. 1938. *Trends in Hospital Development, 1928–1936.* Public Health Bulletin, no. 243, part 2. Washington, DC: USGPO.

Munro, William Bennet. 1923. *Municipal Government and Administration.* Vol. 1. New York: Macmillan.

Muntz, Earl. 1949. *Growth and Trends in Social Security.* Studies in Individual and Collective Security, no. 6. New York: National Conference Board.

Naylor, C. David. 1986. *Private Practice, Public Payment: Canadian Medicine and the Politics of Health Insurance, 1911–1966.* Montreal: McGill-Queen's University Press.

New Brunswick. 1917. *Acts of the Legislative Assembly.* Fredericton: King's Printer.

New York. State Board of Charities. 1900. *Annual Report, 1899.* Vol. 2. Albany: James B. Lyon.

Norman, Vivian. 1952. "Federal Participation in Vendor Payments for Medicare Care." *Social Security Bulletin* 15 (8): 8–10, 21.

Nova Scotia. 1900. *Revised Statutes.* Halifax: Queen's Printer.

Numbers, Ronald L. 1982. "The Specter of Socialized Medicine: American Medicine and Compulsory Health Insurance." In *Compulsory Health Insurance: The Continuing American Debate,* edited by Ronald L. Numbers, 3–24. Westport, CT: Greenwood.

Ontario. 1874. *Revised Statutes.* Toronto: King's Printer.

———. 1914. *Revised Statutes.* Toronto: King's Printer.

———. 1938. *Statement of the Government of Ontario to the Royal Commission on Dominion-Provincial Relations.* Book 3. Toronto: King's Printer.

———. 1950. *Revised Statutes.* Toronto: King's Printer.

———. 1956. *Ontario White Paper (on Hospital Insurance).* Mimeographed.

Ontario. Inspector of Prisons and Public Charities of the Province of Ontario. 1875–1930. *Annual Report.* Sessional Papers. Toronto: King's Printer.

Ontario. Standing Committee on Health. 1956. *Report of Meetings with Respect to Hospital Insurance in Ontario.* Toronto: Queen's Printer.

Pennell, Elliot H., Joseph W. Mountin, and Emily Hankla. 1938. "Summary Figures on Income, Expenditures, and Personnel of Hospitals." *Hospitals* 12 (4): 11–19.

Perry, J. Harvey. 1955. *Taxes, Tariffs, and Subsidies: A History of Canadian Fiscal Development.* Vol. 2. Toronto: University of Toronto Press.

Pilcher, Louis S. 1890. "The Public Hospitals of Brooklyn." *Proceedings of the National Conference of Charities and Corrections* 17:177–89.

Poen, Monte M. 1979. *Harry S. Truman versus the Medical Lobby: The Genesis of Medicare.* Columbia, MO: University of Columbia Press.

Quebec. 1925. *Revised Statutes.* Quebec: King's Printer.

Quebec. Bureau of Statistics. 1914–40. *Statistical Yearbook.* Quebec: King's Printer.

Reed, Louis. 1964. "Private Consumer Expenditures for Medical Care and Voluntary Health Insurance, 1948–63." *Social Security Bulletin* 27 (12): 12–22.

———. 1967. "Private Health Insurance: Coverage and Financial Experience, 1940–66." *Social Security Bulletin* 30 (11): 3–22.

Rorem, C. Rufus. 1934. "Policies and Procedures for Group Hospitalization." *Bulletin of the American Hospital Association* 8 (5): 9–12.

Rosenberg, Charles. 1987. *The Care of Strangers: The Rise of America's Hospital System.* New York: Basic Books.

Rothman, David. 1971. *The Discovery of the Asylum: Social Order and Disorder in the New Republic.* Boston: Little, Brown.

Saskatchewan. 1909. *Revised Statutes.* Regina: King's Printer.

———. 1920. *Revised Statutes.* Regina: King's Printer.

Saskatchewan. Department of Public Health. 1938. *Annual Report, 1936.* Sessional Papers. Regina: King's Printer.

Schneider, David M. 1938. *The History of Public Welfare in New York State, 1609–1866.* Chicago: University of Chicago Press.

Schneider, David M., and Albert Deutsch. 1941. *The History of Public Welfare in New York State, 1867–1940.* Chicago: University of Chicago Press.

Seavoy, Ronald. 1982. *The Origins of the American Business Corporation, 1784–1855.* Westport, CT: Greenwood.

Short, Adam, and Arthur Doughty. 1914. *Canada and Its Provinces.* Vol. 18. Toronto: Publisher's Association.

Skocpol, Theda. 1992. *Protecting Soldiers and Mothers: The Political Origins of Social Policy in the United States.* Cambridge, MA: Belknap Press, Harvard University Press.

Somers, Herman. 1968. "Medicare and the Cost of Health Services." In *The American System of Social Insurance: Its Philosophy, Impact, and Future Development,* edited by William G. Bowen et al., 119–43. New York: McGraw-Hill.

Splane, Richard. 1968. *Social Welfare in Ontario, 1791–1893: A Study in Public Welfare Administration.* Toronto: University of Toronto Press.

Starr, Paul. 1982. *The Social Transformation of American Medicine.* New York: Basic Books.

Stevens, Robert, and Rosemary Stevens. 1974. *Welfare Medicine in America: A Case Study of Medicaid.* New York: Free Press.

Stevens, Rosemary. 1984. "Sweet Charity: State Aid to Hospitals in Pennsylvania, 1870–1910." *Bulletin of the History of Medicine* 58:287–314, 474–95.

———. 1989. *In Sickness and in Wealth: American Hospitals in the Twentieth Century.* New York: Basic Books.

Stewart, Gordon T. 1986. *The Origin of Canadian Politics: A Comparative Approach.* Vancouver: University of British Columbia Press.

Sturges, Gertrude. 1944. "Medical Services under Public Welfare Departments: Some Recent Advances." *Medical Care* 4 (3): 206–11.

Swidler, Ann. 1986. "Culture in Action: Symbols and Strategies." *American Sociological Review* 51:273–86.

Taylor, Malcolm G. 1987. *Health Insurance and Canadian Public Policy.* 2d ed. Montreal: McGill-Queen's University Press.

Thelen, Kathleen, and Sven Steinmo. 1992. "Historical Institutionalism in Comparative Politics." In *Structuring Politics: Historical Institutionalism in Comparative Analysis,* edited by Sven Steinmo, Kathleen Thelen, and Frank Longstreth, 1–32. New York: Cambridge University Press.

Trattner, Walter I. 1984. *From Poor Law to Welfare State: A History of Social Welfare in America.* New York: Free Press.

U.S. Bureau of the Census. 1905. *Benevolent Institutions, 1904.* Washington, DC: USGPO.

———. 1913. *Benevolent Institutions, 1910.* Washington, DC: USGPO.

———. 1914. *Summary of State Laws Relating to the Dependent Classes, 1913.* Washington, DC: USGPO.

———. 1925. *Hospitals and Dispensaries, 1923.* Washington, DC: USGPO.

———. 1975. *Historical Statistics of the United States: Colonial Times to 1970.* Part 1. Washington, DC: USGPO.

U.S. Commission on Intergovernmental Relations. 1955. *A Report to the President for Transmittal to Congress.* Washington, DC: USGPO.

U.S. Department of Health, Education and Welfare. 1958. *Health Insurance and Related Proposals for Financing Personal Health Services: A Digest,* by Agnes Brewster. Washington, DC: USGPO.

———. 1960. *Principles for Planning the Future Hospital System: A Report of the Proceedings of Four Regional Conferences.* Public Health Service, publication no. 721. Washington, DC: USGPO.

U.S. Department of Labor. 1949. *Workmen's Compensation Problems, 1949.* Bulletin no. 119. Washington, DC: USGPO.

U.S. Interdepartmental Committee to Coordinate Health and Welfare Activities. 1938. *Proceedings of the National Health Conference, July 18, 19, 20, 1938.* Washington, DC: USGPO.

U.S. Senate Committee on Education and Labor. 1939. *To Establish a National Health Program: Hearings on S. 1620.* 76th Cong., 1st sess., pt. 2.

———. 1946. *National Health Program: Hearings on S. 1606.* 79th Cong., 2nd sess., pt. 3.

U.S. Senate Subcommittee of the Committee on Labor and Public Welfare. 1949. *National Health Program, 1949: Hearings on S. 1106, S. 1456, S. 1581, and S. 1679.* 81st Cong., 1st sess., pt. 1.

Warner, Amos, et al. 1935. *American Charities and Social Work.* 4th ed. New York: Thomas Cromwell.

White, Ruth. 1952a. "Expenditures for Medical Services in Public Assistance, 1946." *Social Security Bulletin* 15 (9): 7–12, 20.

———. 1952b. *Medical Care in Public Assistance, 1946.* Public Assistance Report no. 18, part 2, *Summary Report.* Washington, DC: Federal Security Agency.

Index